INTRODUCING EXISTENTIAL HEALTH

Introducing Existential Health unfolds this evolving concept and places it in the context of common understandings of health. It presents existential health as a vital dimension in understanding human well-being, complementing the traditional biopsychosocial model. It critiques reductionist and mechanistic views of health and showcases a new four-dimensional model in healthcare practice and design that integrates biological, psychological, social, and existential dimensions. Presented as a valid alternative to the biopsychosocial model, it provides modern system thinking and a holistic understanding centred around meaning and the first-person perspective to give a voice to intersectional discourses and encourage equality in health.

The book traces the historical evolution of health understandings, highlighting the gaps in addressing subjective and existential perspectives. It examines existential health through various lenses, including meaning-making, subjective experiences, and empirical correlations with other dimensions of health. Practical applications are discussed, emphasising the role of existential health in prevention, chronic disease management, and end-of-life care. The book also advocates for educational reforms to include training in existential health approaches and holistic care. By enriching the language and frameworks for existential health, this book aims to inspire a cultural shift in healthcare towards a more integrative and person-centred paradigm.

The book is intended for all health professionals interested in the quality of healthcare in modern society and for health education. The models presented in the book are of a heuristic nature, suitable for reflection, discussion, and teaching about health. It is also valuable reading for researchers in academic health professions and those in the development of health politics, searching for arguments and stepping stones for a more holistic health perspective.

Peter la Cour is from Denmark, works as a clinical health psychologist, and holds a time-limited position as professor adjunct at MF, Oslo Norway. His PhD was in psychology of religion, and he been a part of a Norwegian research network now called "Research center for existential health" for the past 15 years.

INTRODUCING EXISTENTIAL HEALTH

The Four-Dimensional Model

Peter la Cour

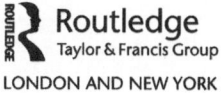

Routledge
Taylor & Francis Group

LONDON AND NEW YORK

Designed cover image: getty images via sesame

First published 2025
by Routledge
4 Park Square, Milton Park, Abingdon, Oxon OX14 4RN

and by Routledge
605 Third Avenue, New York, NY 10158

Routledge is an imprint of the Taylor & Francis Group, an informa business

British Library Cataloguing-in-Publication Data
A catalogue record for this book is available from the British Library

ISBN: 9781032819877 (hbk)
ISBN: 9781032818511 (pbk)
ISBN: 9781003502364 (ebk)

DOI: 10.4324/9781003502364

Typeset in Times New Roman
by Newgen Publishing UK

Access the Support Material: www.routledge.com/9781003502364

CONTENTS

Preface   *vii*

PART I
The four-dimensional model   **1**

1 History of health understandings and definitions   3
   1.1 The lost sense of wholeness 3
   1.2 The WHO's history of defining health 7
   1.3 The lack of consensus in definitions of physical,
   *   psychological, and social health 11*

2 The biopsychosocial model and the critique   18
   2.1 Presentation of the biopsychosocial model (BPS) 18
   2.2 Early critique: What BPS is and isn't 20
   2.3 Later critique of the BPS model 24
   2.4 The general lack of first-person perspectives in medicine 30

3 Background for a restructured model   32
   3.1 The need for a new model 32
   3.2 Illness causality and systems theory imagery 37
   3.3 Subjectivity, health, and lifeworlds 40

4 The four-dimensional model of health and illness 46
    4.1 Characteristics of the four dimensions one by one 46
    4.2 Limitations and abilities of the four-dimensional model 51

PART II
What is existential health? **53**

5 Explorations in existential health 55
    5.1 What makes a topic existential? 55
    5.2 Existential health definitions 59

6 Mapping the terrain of existential health 68
    6.1 Categories of components in existential health 69

7 Empirical connections: Existential health and other health
   dimensions 75
    7.1 Existential expressions and health correlates 76
    7.2 Existential qualities and health correlates 81
    7.3 Life orientations and health correlates 85
    7.4 Subjective experience of living and health correlates 87

8 Where the presence of existential health is already evident 90
    8.1 Examples of relevant existential health concerns
       during the lifespan 90
    8.2 Prevention of illness and existential health 95

9 Some implications of existential health 98
    9.1 Training 100
    9.2 'Physician, heal thyself' 101

10 Epilogue 103

References *105*
Index *117*

PREFACE

My first job after graduating in psychology was a one-year training position at the psychiatric unit of the National Hospital in Denmark. The head psychologist there was also responsible for a full course in psychology for medical students at the University of Copenhagen. One day she found herself short of teachers, and I was interested. My subsequent professional positions have been very varied, mostly in health psychology and research, but somehow teaching at medical school has always followed.

For a long time, the teaching in medically oriented psychology was organised together with the unit for general practice, and the biopsychosocial model was one of the topics. In the beginning, the teaching of the biopsychosocial model was very enthusiastic; it was a model that fitted well with the attitudes of general practice. As the years went by, the main lecture on the topic somehow ended up at my desk, and preparing the lecture semester after semester soon became more and more problematic for me. It seemed like a lot of hot air. Reading about it just reinforced the feeling of many good intentions and not much more. The lecture evolved as more and more critical towards the model – not the intentions – which annoyed the general practice colleagues. They very much wanted the model to show their uniqueness as the discipline with the most holistic views of patients, which may be true. My problem was that the model itself was difficult to talk about in a coherent way. The critical thoughts were fed by reading articles, not really research but commentaries and theoretical inputs in journals, and discussing things in the lectures. General practice was not happy with that development.

I started to rearrange the model to make it more logical and comprehensive. In my computer files, I found the first PowerPoint presentation with the existential seen as part of health dating back to 2012. Since then the subject of this book has been on the move, constantly changing a little bit here and there and with a growing interest in the concept of existential health itself. At some point, the continuing adjustments have to harden, usually when things are written down and published. The first manuscript about the rethinking of the model dates back more than six years back.

It is a difficult field to navigate because there are so many interests and viewpoints already present. On the one hand, there are interests that want to hold on to the very simplified understanding of the biopsychosocial model as a model for holistic medicine, and on the other hand, there are biomedical interests that will only accept evidence from randomised trials as relevant medical knowledge. The topic seems to provoke quite strong and very different reactions, no matter where I presented the thoughts.

Then I decided to write this book, and it has been a pleasure cruise ever since. A very kind publisher showed interest in it a year ago, and the ideas have continued to be supported by dear colleagues, of whom I thank Professor Lars Johan Danbolt for his fundamental trust in my work throughout, and in particular, I thank Professor Tatjana Schnell for her continuing inspiration, partnership and know-how.

Times have also changed and may now be more ripe for thinking about existential health. In 2024, the Swedish government commissioned the Public Health Agency to assess the possibilities of integrating existential health into Sweden's public health efforts. And in academic journals we can read a text like this:

> In a highly medicalized society, we need to reinvent our language for the existential struggles, and the suffering that always accompanies them. If a concept of 'existential health' can make us more aware of the fact that the existential concerns are always a part of both health and illness, it is worth developing. Klik eller tryk her for at skrive tekst.
>
> *(Binder, 2022)*

I hope that this book will be an inspiration to the reader for further reflections about health and existence.

Peter la Cour
December 2024

PART I
The four-dimensional model

1

HISTORY OF HEALTH UNDERSTANDINGS AND DEFINITIONS

1.1 The lost sense of wholeness

Health and methods of improving health seem to be interwoven through evolution. Health equals survival and life unfolded, and the line between automatic evolutionary strategies for survival and the use of remedies for self-medication is very thin. Some parrots and other animals are known to eat clay to aid digestion and kill bacteria. More evolved animals, such as the great apes, deliberately seek out and eat specific plants, usually outside their diet, which appear to serve specific functions in coping with parasites (Fruth et al., 2014; Neco et al., 2019). Such behaviour is known in biology as self-medication.

We do not know how to define the transition from animal to human. Some of the best distinctions might not be deliberate tool-making and use or the evidence of self-awareness, as has been suggested in the past since many of the higher animals have been shown to use tools in an advanced way and to be able to recognise themselves in mirrors.

Evidence of group care for the sick is found from early in human evolution but is most evident among the Neanderthals, where skulls with disabling, but healed fractures are often found. The individuals could not have survived or healed without live-sustaining efforts of the group or family. It is also clear from the healed bones that the care must have included the use of antibacterial plants (Hardy, 2021).

This caring could be suggested as distinct human behaviour, but at some later point in history, more defining signs of humanity appear. This is something new in evolution, namely the habit of greeting the dead by burying them with grave gifts – suggesting a belief in a world differing from this, the world of the spirit. At the same time, signs of rituals, including traces of paint, are found in the remains and in jewellery such as beads and shells.

DOI: 10.4324/9781003502364-2

Deliberate burials and the use of paint are found even among the Neanderthals (Balzeau et al., 2020), but remnants of advanced human cognition and culture are much easier to recognise from the Stone Age, defined by the 'big bang of human culture,' also called the cognitive revolution around 50,000 years ago (Hatfield & Pittman, 2013). From there, elements of a human society can be pieced together, and ideas about the health of humans can be traced.

As far as we know, there seemed to be very few differences in various kinds of suffering. Physical illness, mental difficulties, the survival of the tribe, and relations with the spirit world were probably perceived as closely interwoven, almost as one and the same thing. If a person had difficulties, they could go to the shaman, and the tradition of the shaman can be witnessed and traced in cave art and other remains (Clottes & Lewis-Williams, 1998). The shaman was a universalist and took care of everything: physical illness, mental problems, the social well-being of the tribe, and keeping peace with the spirits. The shaman was probably not the leader of the tribe, but an authority alongside leadership. The shaman was – in modern terms – a combination of a physician, psychologist, social worker, and priest. All four functions might be found in the picture of a shaman from the Trois Frere cave from around 15,000 years BCE (Figure 1.1).

Since then, this original wholeness has been divided and separated into different areas of recognition. Without precise dating, we can trace some of the steps. Plato philosophises about the nature of the soul around 500 BCE. He argues that the soul has an existence which is different from that of the body. The soul has its own project; the body and the soul each have their own logic. Body and soul are seen as separate things. The Greek physician Galen built a medical science and practice around the theory of the body: it has four bodily fluids: yellow bile and black bile, mucus, and blood, and the body has thus acquired its own material dimension with associated medical practitioners of the profession (Koenig et al., 2012).

In the Western cultural context, medical thinking grows out of this. In the first centuries of the Christian context, however, the four bodily fluids did not have much influence. Illness had other roots. It was understood mainly as a response to sin, like in the Old Testament, and the cure for illness was to restore the right relationship with God. In the Old Testament, making offerings in the temple was the remedy; in early Christianity, praying and repentance were the main remedies. The care for the sick took place in monastery-like environments, and Christian physicians usually had basic theological education. Medicine was a subdivision of religious knowledge, and physicians, like priests, were all men. A new development occurred in the fourth century when the founding father Augustine recognised that medicine was a profession in its own right, independent of theology, thus giving space to women as competent in the function of midwives (Koenig et al., 2012; Porter, 2003). In early monastic history, theology-based care also provided space for the development of medical techniques and plant-based medicines and for medical curiosity, including knowledge of anatomy.

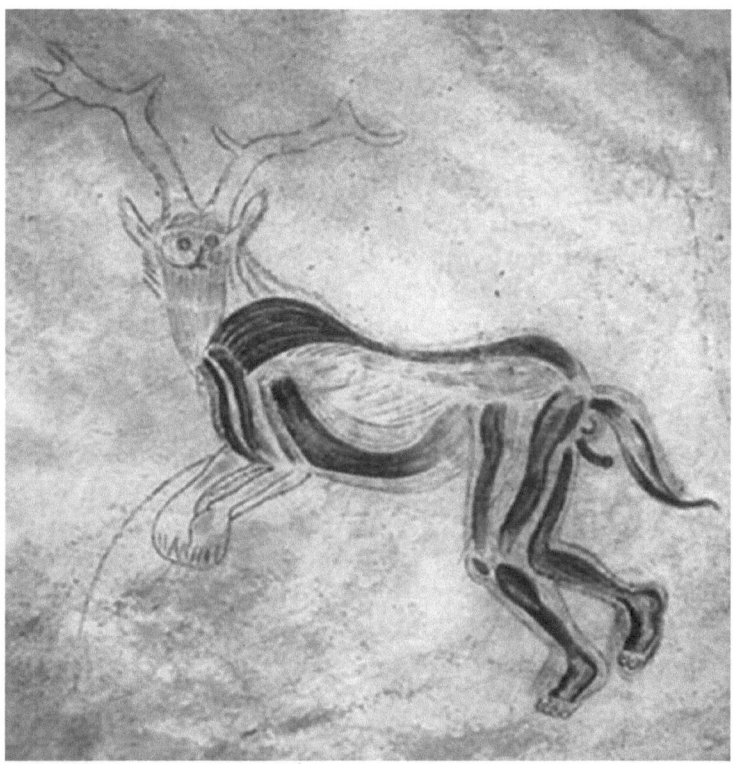

FIGURE 1.1   The shaman had multiple knowledge and functions. Cave painting from the Trois Frere Cave in France, c. 15,000 years BCE.

The dead body, the corps, remained sacrosanct until the years up to 1600, when the church allowed fresh corpses to be dissected for anatomical studies. It became clear that the blood flowed around the body and was not stationary, as the theory of body fluids and the technique of vein loading had assumed. The philosopher Descartes declared that there was no place where the soul could have materially resided in the dead bodies, and he theorised that the body and the soul consisted of two different substances, *res extensa* and *res cogitans*. Body and soul were now completely separate – a fundamental dualism was a reality in Western thought.

In the history of medicine, mental disorders first appear clearly as identities with neurology and psychiatry around the year 1900. It became clear that mental illness was not primarily due to bad morals and depraved lifestyles, but could have neurological as well as psychological causes. It was no longer necessary to have moral teachings of conduct and thought life in psychiatry, and a distinction was drawn between the psychological and the spiritual/theological. We now have the division of health into three realms (body, mind, soul), and we have three learned professions that could all take care of the suffering human: the doctor, the psychiatrist (psychologist), and the priest (Koenig et al., 2012).

In the latter half of the twentieth century, a yet new medical field became independent due to the increased understanding of the social and societal dimensions of health. Public health was established as a new health discipline. At this point in time, it was technically possible to be able to handle larger amounts of data, and it became clear that individuals got sick and died not only as individuals but as parts of groups and societies. Environment, social conditions, social possibilities, and economics make people sick and healthy, independent of the individual's point of view and the abilities of the medical profession. As something new, medical science can function without involving the individual patient. Social and environmental medicine becomes the fourth division of health in a modern perspective.

In this way, human health is no longer a unified object of study, even though the word health originates from *helthe* = wholeness, a being whole, sound, or well, (with associations also to holy, sacred, and to heal).

Contemporary human health has been divided into four independently understood dimensions. In modern terms, we could call the dimensions biological,

TABLE 1.1 The lost wholeness

Approx dating	*Organisation*	*Dimensions*
Before 2000 BCE	Shamans: Priest/physician/psychologist	No division
2000 BCE	Old Testament medicine is supernatural medicine	No division
600 BCE	Medicine emerges as a profession with Hippocrates Plato singles out the soul as a special entity	Body and soul
100 CE	Early Christianity: illness answers sin. Prayer heals – there is no difference between the soul, the body or the spirit	No division
400 CE	Augustine recognises specially trained, secularly knowledgeable 'medicine persons' (midwives)	Medicine without theology
1400 CE	Clashes between religion and medicine	Religion versus science
1700 CE	Descartes: The body becomes truly secular and godless. The body is separated from the immortal soul	Body and soul
1900 CE	Psychology arises – the doctrine of mental illnesses seen as purely secular	Body Mind differs from soul
1920 CE	Karl Barth: The psyche is completely separated from the divine	Religion without psychology
1980 CE	Public Health/Social Medicine: The social is separated from the individual (social medicine)	Biostatistics

psychological, environmental/social, and existential. All four dimensions are very difficult to accommodate at once, and the question arises of how we can withhold any understanding of human life, health, and well-being as a whole.

This becomes a problem in the everyday life of any clinical health worker, where the clinician is facing and relating to a patient in a consultation. The patient is only one and the same; the patient is not divided into different parts and areas in the real world.

1.2 The WHO's history of defining health

1.2.1 Health as well-being

After the calamities of the two world wars, a broad movement among politicians reacted with the aspiration that world wars should never happen again. The vision behind the creation of the United Nations in 1945 was huge. It was a vision of a better world, and health was an important part of the greater good. The Health Department of the United Nations, WHO, was funded in 1948 and had a very broad scope of serving mankind by promoting 'health for all' (Peng-Keller et al., 2022). It was not called 'international health' but 'world health,' and the target was nothing less than health for the whole world.

But what did they mean by the word 'health'? The main perspective was a kind of public health in a very broad sense, total health for everyone, everywhere, thereby taking a distance to the narrow Western medical paradigm, and lifting the scope from doctor–patient relations to a cross-cultural formulation.

In the constitutional preamble for the WHO from 1948 the first two bullet points are:

- Health is a state of complete physical, mental and social well-being and not merely the absence of disease or infirmity.
- The enjoyment of the highest attainable standard of health is one of the fundamental rights of every human being without distinction of race, religion, political belief, economic or social condition.

By these sentences, health is understood in a very broad and holistic way, and it connects health to human rights and to a social and political agenda.

However, *holism* is not a well-defined concept. In the works of medical historian Charles Rosenberg (Freeman, 2005; Peng-Keller et al., 2022), holism in medicine can be distinguished into at least four types: 1) Historical holism, concerning the ancient ways of medical thinking and holistic healing (named 'the lost whole' above); 2) Organismic holism, aiming at unifying the body and mind; 3) Ecological holism, where organisms are seen embedded in their environment; 4) Ideological holism, in which health and healing are connected to the social and the society. The WHO ideas about holism seem best to be covered by the category of ideological holism.

In the WHO 1948 definition of health, the word 'well-being' seems to be the most important concept, and the words 'more than the absence of disease' seem to be the most borderless phrase.

There is no definition of well-being offered anywhere by the WHO, and this lack of definition is almost always the case in texts concerning health (Jarden & Roache, 2023). The concept of well-being has been central across many academic disciplines at least since the Greek philosophers, who divided and discussed individual contentment with life in terms of hedonistic versus eudaimonic well-being, which could be translated as pleasure versus meaningfulness as the basis of well-being (Disabato et al., 2016). In a recent overview of the term 'well-being,' it is usually defined by words with nearly the same meaning, such as 'how well one's life is going' or 'a state of happiness and contentment [...] overall good physical and mental health and outlook, or good quality of life' (Jarden & Roache, 2023). According to the same authors, a widely used and cited definition of well-being goes like this: 'Well-being can be understood as how people feel and how they function both on a personal and social level and how they evaluate their lives as a whole' (Michaelson et al., 2012, p. 6).

It might be notable from modern reflections on the word 'well-being' that there is very little emphasis on physical health and that the notions of 'quality and evaluation of life' are central. In health, this notion seems to be in contrast to the overwhelming dominance of biomedicine perspectives in modern Western health. Biomedical thinking has the power in medical theory, research, research funding, medical industry and economy, the world of health insurance, social welfare systems, health policy, and health administration. The WHO definition of health as well-being seems simply very little reflected in modern health understandings.

1.2.2 Health as more than bio, psycho, and social?

The WHO preamble of 1948 stated physical, mental, and social as the dimensions of well-being, but this division into three dimensions did not have much impact on Western healthcare, at least until it was reformulated as the biopsychosocial model by Georg L. Engel 20 years later (Engel, 1977).

The WHO definition of health was again the subject of a WHO meeting in 1983. There was a growing dissatisfaction with the naming of the three dimensions of bio, psycho, and social, especially in Eastern and African cultures, where well-being was seen as closely associated with something internal and higher, connected to the joy and to the appreciation of living. In some of these cultures, this highly missing dimension was best coined as 'spiritual.'

In a recent book titled *The Spirit of Global Health* (Peng-Keller et al., 2022), the historical documents and debate around the 36th World Health Assembly in 1983, are summarised in an extended way. The health minister of Swaziland is cited with this statement from the meeting:

there is a dimension to a man or a woman that goes beyond and above his physical, mental and social well-being. There is something within the person [...] what one could call attitude, motivation, driving force, or whatever name you wish to call it or define it, but which I prefer to call spirit.

(Peng-Keller et al., 2022, p. 45)

He was not alone. Several attempts to add the 'spiritual dimension' to the concluding papers from the conference were made, and the debate is described as intense. There was a suggestion to change the wording of the constitution to: 'Health is a state of complete physical, mental, social and spiritual well-being.'

The opposite side of the debate was not against the idea of adding a new dimension of health, but they did not understand what the meaning of the words in the spiritual dimension was really about. They then debated the words, trying to describe what was meant by 'spiritual.' No consensus was reached. The relationship between religion and spirituality was discussed, and there were arguments for a general broader understanding, including mental health, medical ethics, respect for people's culture, health education, and other issues (Peng-Keller et al., 2022, p. 51).

At the meeting the year after, the topic of spiritual health was taken up again, but the text with the additional dimension of health was voted down. The concept spiritual was found too unclear.

Nevertheless, the term 'spirituality' sneaked in again into the WHO papers on health in 1989, where the term 'spiritual care' was found essential in relation to palliation and end-of-life care.

The fuzziness of the word 'spirituality' has been noted several times since. In 2006, it was observed from a religious viewpoint that the measurement of spirituality in medicine often included questions about psychological well-being, satisfaction, connectedness with others, hopefulness, meaning and purpose in life, and altruistic values. These questions are either determined as tautological for general health (asking the same question in different versions twice) or as tapping indicators of mental health, and thereby meaningless as a separate dimension (Moreira-Almeida & Koenig, 2006b)

In 2012, a study of the understanding of 'spirituality' in a secular setting found six quite different understandings and uses of the word (la Cour et al., 2012).

In a serious recent attempt to reinstall 'spiritual' to health in the book mentioned above, it is suggested that spiritual is 1) a depth dimension of health that 2) calls for interprofessional collaboration, respecting 3) spiritual plurality to make it 4) an evaluative concept (Peng-Keller et al., 2022).

In spite of these attempts to retain something essential for health, that is not captured in the bio, psycho, and social dimensions, the word 'spiritual' simply seems to be a poor choice of wording, as it originates from religion and has very different connotations dependent on the religion and culture involved. Although several elements are mentioned as content, there is no constitutional element, making the term 'spiritual' essentially different from the bio, psycho, and social.

1.2.3   Health as a resource

A lot was happening in 1984. The WHO had also set up groups on *health promotion*, an emerging concept in 1984. One group met in Copenhagen. Their topic was to determine what health promotion was and to define their topic, and in doing so, they had to think in a new way. Their starting point was acknowledging that health promotion was about changes in something; it was linked to dynamic processes (WHO, 1984). In seeing health as something dynamic, the old 1948 definition of health as well-being became a problem, as health is defined here as a state of something, something static. Thereby, the conditions and ways of changing health to the worse or the better remained unclear and untold.

Health is heavily dependent on conditions, the group claimed, and basic resources for health are income, shelter, and food. Health promotion involves more than just securing these basics. It also involves supporting things like health information and life skills, services and facilities. In other words, it involves the total environment (WHO, 1984).

Health is something changing and dependent on the surroundings. If good resources are available, good health is possible. Seeing health in such dynamics, the very definition of health is now altered by the group in this way:

> Health [is] [...] the extent to which an individual or group is able to realize aspirations and satisfy needs and to change or cope with the environment. Health is a resource for everyday life, not the objective of living; it is a positive concept, emphasizing social and personal resources, as well as physical capacities.
>
> *(WHO, 1984)*

With this definition, the associations with health have changed. The main concept is now resource, not well-being, and the order of the elements bio, psycho, and social are here changed: On the basis of the *environment*, the social and the psychological are named as resources and come before the physical, which is named a capacity.

According to this definition, people are able to take control of and be responsible for their own health, as long as they have the information, organisation, and 'total environment' to do so.

Health is understood as the capacity for living everyday life, and by that there is an emphasis on *functioning*. There is no notion of being perfect or flawless in any dimension. In fact, it seems that one can be healthy in a quite disabled position, for example as physically handicapped, if the environment is able to contribute with the necessary resources and capacities to 'satisfy needs and to change or cope with the environment.'

The notion of health not being 'the objective of living' points in the same direction. Health does not mean a condition free of disease or disability, as long as these faults and defects do not impair the individual's ability to perform the tasks intended to cope with and change the environment.

Health does not exclude un-health, as long as the dynamics and the functioning of the whole human system suit the purpose of coping and changing. It is a truly positive concept focusing on the abilities, resources, and capabilities of living in the world. Only when health does not represent sufficient resources (physical, mental, or social) can we talk about being in an un-healthy position, which is considered a negative.

Health is no longer tied to the individual; it can be the health of a group. This can give meaning to evolutionary psychology, where groups – tribes – that did not have the necessary resources for survival died as a group. This could be due to a lack of environmental supplies (e.g. food), physical disease (e.g. insufficient immune system), cognitive abilities (e.g. poor visual recognition skills, finding way), or social resources (e.g. group fighting strength in tribal fights).

At an individual level, one can pursue the activities of daily living – and be considered healthy – even without legs, if a wheelchair is functioning; with no eyes, if survival patterns are trained; or with mild stages of dementia, if the family are supportive and can bring joy to life.

This really is a new way of understanding health – and it raises thoughts about life itself and perhaps even death. Perhaps feeling unwell is sometimes part of building up resources for future aspirations and coping?

These dynamic perspectives on health are very welcomed in future concepts of health. They turn away the attention from the overwhelming power of sometimes rather short-sighted and context-missing biomedical thinking.

1.3 The lack of consensus in definitions of physical, psychological, and social health

1.3.1 Physical health

It seems obvious to many that biomedical health is the opposite of biomedical illness. This is shown by laboratory tests. They are not ambiguous; they show whether this blood sample is positive or negative, whether this leg is broken or not, and whether this woman is pregnant or not.

In the real world, every health worker has experienced the opposite. The clinical discussions and energy are dedicated to everything that is not that straightforward. A blood sample is on the border, or insignificant below, somewhat below, or can be above but with no clinical relevance. A bone is broken in a simple or complicated way, and the context is the determining factor for the clinical interventions chosen or left behind. A pregnant woman may be pregnant outside the womb, she may be pregnant with a child with genetic defects, she may be pregnant after a rape. Or she may not be pregnant after seven years of trying to get pregnant.

And what is a physical illness? Are you ill if you are missing a little finger on your left hand? If you are a well-treated and symptom-free asthmatic? If you can't stand being in the sun? If you can't have children? If you do not get an erection every time it is wanted? Nothing is really black and white here.

So, how do we measure health and illness? The most obvious thing might be the length of living. Medical historian Roy Porter (2003) considers the ever-increasing expected lifetime in the Western world as very good news along with the decline in infant mortality. Along with this, the number of medical interventions, such as hip replacements, is ever-growing, and medicine is claimed to do miracles. On the other hand, anxiety about health and the feeling of health dangers everywhere seem also ever-growing, and we are not able to see medicine without a dialectical relationship to mentality, Porter writes. We are healthier, but also without confidence in the doctors and the medical system. Furthermore, the line between physical health and other agendas has become more and more unclear. Porter gives an example of a widow given permission to be pregnant with the semen of her dead husband. Is that a health discussion at all? Is that an answer to a medical problem?

Hardcore biomedical spokesmen might claim that illness and health have only one absolute enemy: death. When a living organism is dead, it is certainly not healthy. But again, we get into trouble because of the circumstances, the context. In all Western countries, we are now discussing euthanasia and active assistance in dying, and passive death help has been around for centuries. Sometimes death is preferable to life.

Beef is defined as good if the animal it was taken from was without disease – but the flesh of the steak is, of course, dead. Death might not be the opposite of physical health.

It gets even more complicated when we try to capture what is meant by health when it is defined as 'more than the absence of illness' – when we have no clear idea of what illness is. And what are the elements of 'more than'? What is 'more than' made of? According to the WHO, well-being is the central element of health, but what does well-being consist of? What is well-being?

It does not get any easier when health is defined as a resource or homeostasis. Here, health is no longer an empirical physical thing, but a quality of living in relation to the surroundings. The surroundings or the environment is not part of the living organism itself and therefore not definable as something biomedically inherent.

1.3.2 Mental health

The idea of health as a resource and of maintaining homeostasis, as suggested by the WHO in 1984, seems to be the key point in the WHO definition of *mental health*. The WHO defined mental health in this way in 2005 (World Health Organization, 2005):

a state of well-being in which the individual realizes his or her abilities, can cope with the normal stresses of life, can work productively and fruitfully, and can contribute to his or her community.

This statement was later paraphrased on several occasions and in several ways; the wording of the definition seems not as authoritative as with previous WHO definitions of health. The extended rephrasing often claims that mental health is 'more than the absence of mental disorders' but also emphasises several other dimensions of life (WHO, 2022). This very open attitude does not really clarify the concept of mental health; it gets really muddy. Included are, for example, the individual's *realising* (self-awareness), the ability to *cope* (psychological functioning), *work productivity* (physical functioning), and *contribution to the community* (social engagement).

An all-encompassing definition is well intentioned but not really helpful in the conceptualisation of what is important, and it makes it nearly impossible to operationalise in an empirical sensible manner like it is wished for in the health systems.

Across definitions, the most common consensus seems to be that mental health is more than the absence of mental disorders. However, mental diseases and their treatment are the main content of chapters on psychological health in many textbooks (Insel et al., 2011), even though they are named 'negative definitions' in the introduction. The disciplines of psychiatry and clinical psychology have dealt with *bad* mental health in Western culture for 150 years. Psychiatric illnesses are now listed in diagnostic manuals such as the *ICD11*, which comprises a continuously updated number of officially labelled psychiatric diseases. Some of these are seen as closely related to body or nerve abnormalities, such as dementia or abuse-related hallucinations, while most conditions are seen and described independently of body and nerve functions, such as personality traits like antisocial personality disorder.

Much less is written about psychologically *good* health. What are the features of good mental health? There is certainly no single answer, but in 1993 American psychologists Daniel Batson, Patricia Schoenrade, and W. Larry Ventis tried to make a list including the following seven different kinds of definitions of mental health (Batson et al., 1993):

Absence of mental illness: The psychiatric perspective that we are healthy in the absence of mental illness (negative definition).
Appropriate social behaviour: The cognitive psychology view of social adjustment as the best sign of mental health (culturally relative).
Freedom from worry and guilt: The psychoanalytic ideal of a truce in the constant inner struggle between conflicting inner forces.
Personal competence and control: The more power-oriented ideals of self-mastery (e.g. Adlerian psychology).
Self-acceptance or self-actualisation: The American humanistic psychology ideals of full personal growth towards some sort kind of completion.
Personality unification and organisation: The ideal of a unique mature balance between personality and environment.

7. *Open-mindedness and flexibility:* The ideology that narrow-minded and rigid persons live less attractive lives.

Seen from a historical perspective, the list contains very ideological statements that were presented at the time as some kind of universals. Especially elderly American values are highlighted – as can be expected from a list developed by American authors in the 1990s.

Moving on to more modern texts of positive definitions, we find headlines such as these defining mental health: realism, acceptance, autonomy, capacity for intimacy, and creativity. Among the psychological tasks to be mastered are: being less defensive, being optimistic, and dealing with anger (Insel et al., 2011). It would not be too hard to bring such a list of positive psychological abilities more up to date by adding the buzzwords of the contemporary and modern psychotherapeutic movements. Concepts such as 'mindful,' 'resilience,' and 'commitment' might capture some dominant psychotherapeutic ideals in contemporary Western psychology.

These kinds of lists can be expanded in multiple ways, and they show that psychological health can be seen, and has been seen, in an ideological and culturally malleable way, deeply related to societal context and contemporary cultural values.

However, something else is striking and noteworthy about the definitions and lists. Some of the qualities mentioned look at psychological health from the *outside*, as observable (e.g. social adaptation), while others see psychological health from the *inside* (e.g. self-acceptance). This might look like a detail, but it hides a big and old schism in the field of psychology.

1.3.2.1   The two kinds of 'mental'

Academic psychology as a discipline has developed along two distinct lines, sometimes referred to as the ideographic and the nomothetic perspectives on the psyche. Historically, this division of psychology originated in the two schools of Wilhelm Wundt and of William James (Hergenhahn, 1997), but this division merely mirrored older dichotomies in theology, philosophy, and the theory of science in general. It is a question of ontology and epistemology (the question of what is true and real, and the principles of how one can know it and how to find out about it.)

Ideographic perspectives take the subjective experience seriously and see the conscious experience as the basis of knowledge of the psyche. The experience of being aware of something and realising something is always individual, private, and unique. Obvious subjective phenomena are, for example, the perception of art, night dreams, existential concerns, and attitudes. Ideographic perspectives focus on the *private* inner life and are less observant of what is given by context, biology, conditions, or other building blocks of the inner psychological life.

Nomothetic perspectives focus on the foundations of psychological life as valid knowledge of the psyche. They acknowledge as valid psychological phenomena that are observable and general, shared between individuals in the *collective* shared world. They view psychology as learning biology and principles; brain and brain functions are central knowledge. The perspective is on what we as biological human beings (brains) have learned from our cultural and physical surroundings and social givens: our learning abilities, our language, norms, social life, socio-ecology, and socio-economics. The psyche also expresses itself in ways open to others and observable, but not usually present for the subject: personality traits, intelligence, and patterns of behaviour. Nomothetic perspectives tend to be less observant of the psychic inner life that cannot be objectified and shared.

The two very different types of psychology are also known as the humanistic and the cognitive/behavioural science perspectives of inner life. They could represent the self seen as the knower ('I,' ideographic) and the self seen as the known ('me,' nomothetic). For decades, these two traditions have lived and competed in academic psychology at universities, as well as in more popular folk psychology thinking. These two different perspectives may live under the same roof, but they are fundamentally quite different dimensions in psychology and everywhere else.

1.3.3   Social health

Contrary to what might be common expectations, there is no united concept of social health. You cannot look it up or Google it as a stand-alone term. A concept of *social capital* has been developed and elaborated over decades, but still a meaningful definition is lacking, along with ways of measuring it (Claridge, 2020).

Usually, social capital is perceived by bringing some other social concepts together. One dictionary lookup could show social capital defined as 'the networks of relationships among people who live and work in a particular society, enabling that society to function effectively' (Dictionary.com), but further elaboration includes a multitude of different topics such as social groups, interpersonal relationships, identity, norms and values, corporations, property, public goods, strategic alliances, and communities. The borders to social determinants, social injustice, and social politics are blurry, and there is no clear line.

Furthermore, social capital is also related to the environment in general (Pretty & Ward, 2001), as the management of natural resources involves collective action – for example, access to water, forestry, agriculture, pesticide control, and so forth. Human interaction with the environment in the form of technology, attitudes, and policies could also be included, named and defined as social capital.

Another understanding of social health could be the umbrella term 'public health,' which in turn also lacks a firm definition, but it is concerned with the measurable health variables of larger groups. It is traditionally defined as 'the science and art of preventing disease, prolonging life and promoting health through the organized efforts and informed choices of society, organizations, public and private, communities and individuals' (Gatseva & Argirova, 2011, p. 205), and is concerned about topics such as group longevity, obesity, tobacco and drinking habits, nutrition, and the like. Climate change brings the relationship between environment and public health very close:

> Climate change is impacting human lives and health in a variety of ways. It threatens the essential ingredients of good health – clean air, safe drinking water, nutritious food supply, and safe shelter – and has the potential to undermine decades of progress in global health.
>
> *(WHO, 2024)*

The lines between network health, social health (social capital), public health, and environmental health appear thin as the topics are highly interconnected. Seen from the individual health perspective, as in a clinical situation, the conceptual lines might not matter much, as it can be described as 'the individual's health relation to the outside world.'

1.3.4 On health definitions

It may come as a surprise that our everyday assumptions about health and healthcare do not rest on solid pillars but rather on feet of clay. Especially in times when evidence-based attitudes appear in almost any health discussion and health decision, it might seem strange that we do not really know or even agree about the very fundamentals of the field. What does it mean, when a person says 'healthy'? What does it mean when a doctor claims 'disease'? It could be like Saint Augustine said about time: If no one asks me, I know what it is. If I wish to explain it to him who asks, I do not know.

Acknowledging a basic human non-knowledge of the basics of the world in which we navigate could presumably lead to a very humble and, thereby, also a very open attitude towards reconsiderations and changes in the field of health, but the opposite seems to be a normal reaction. Not knowing what health is exactly, society in general and medical science in particular are not very open to discussing the limits of knowledge or new findings. It then tends to cling to what is already present, which is the contemporary societal organisation of the healthcare system.

In that way, we mix up the concept of health with the existing health organisations and existing health education, as if they hold the truth about health. That might not be the case, or to be more precise, it probably is not the case. From a perspective above, everybody knows that these matters have always been historically changed, largely influenced by culture, and will probably continue to do so.

There is nothing wrong with a pragmatic attitude towards matters we cannot fully understand. We have to deal with many things we do not understand in everyday life, especially the more fundamental ones – time, for example, as mentioned above, but also our mere existence in an incomprehensible cosmos; the brutal, inexplicable fact that we are here, alive, not knowing how. We have to recognise and embrace a pragmatic attitude to be able to act in the real world.

Being pragmatic, there might be good reasons for reconsideration of the existing order in health organisations in modern Western societies. Do they serve their purpose in a functional way? Are the aims of 'health for all' purposefully mirrored in our health organisation, education, and understanding of healthcare?

There are economic, political, technical, and clinical questions about that. All these domains of thinking need a proper and broad understanding of health in order not to leave the field to the blind forces of biomedical, mechanical thinking and the jungle law of the 'market,' where health is seen from the perspective of economic profit. There is certainly more to human health than that.

2

THE BIOPSYCHOSOCIAL MODEL AND THE CRITIQUE

2.1 Presentation of the biopsychosocial model (BPS)

The WHO claim of health as a biopsychosocial unit became a reality in medical thinking through the works of internist Georg L. Engel in two famous articles from 1977 and 1980. Engel has a clear agenda: he wants to challenge reductionism as the 'dominant dogma' in medicine (Engel, 1977, 1980). He was deeply influenced by psychoanalytic theory and the theories of psychosomatics of the time and viewed ulcerative colitis, for example, as the result of 'strong conscious or unconscious aggressive and sadistic impulses' (Ghaemi, 2010, p. 40).

Engel's two articles are quite different. The first is mainly theoretical and was published in the journal *Science* (Engel, 1977), targeting a general medical audience. Most of the article confronts biomedical thinking and the biological tendencies in psychiatry in the 1970s. Engel argues for multidimensional thinking in health, and he simply mentions the psychological and the social as dimensions involved in health. Some patients feel sick but are well in a medical sense, and some patients are sick in a medical sense but feel well. The psychological and the social aspects must be taken as a key to all illness, he argues. He gives diabetes and schizophrenia as illness examples with obvious psychological and social dimensions, but he makes no actual attempt to build a model, except for naming his proposed multidimensional understanding as the biopsychosocial model (BPS) model. It might be noteworthy that there is no drawing or model of three overlapping circles with words of bio, psycho, and social appearing on them anywhere in the original articles.

The second article was published in the *American Journal of Psychiatry* and was written for psychiatry audiences. It is intended as a clinical application of what is now named the biopsychosocial model, but the article starts with a long

DOI: 10.4324/9781003502364-3

review of the 'general systems theory.' The general systems theory is accredited to biological thinkers from the 1940s (P. A. Weiss and L. von Bertalanffy), and it was developed in reaction to reductionist principles of taking the part out of its context and not recognising the complexity of living systems. A 'system' can be described by its structure, function, and role in relation to other systems, and the systems are placed in a hierarchy of systems, that is, levels of nature building on each other in a bottom-up oriented relationship. This hierarchy of natural systems is depicted by Engel as in Figure 2.1. As seen, the hierarchy goes from 'subatomic particles' to 'biosphere,' but Engel focuses on the levels from 'cells organelles' and to 'community,' which seems most relevant to the

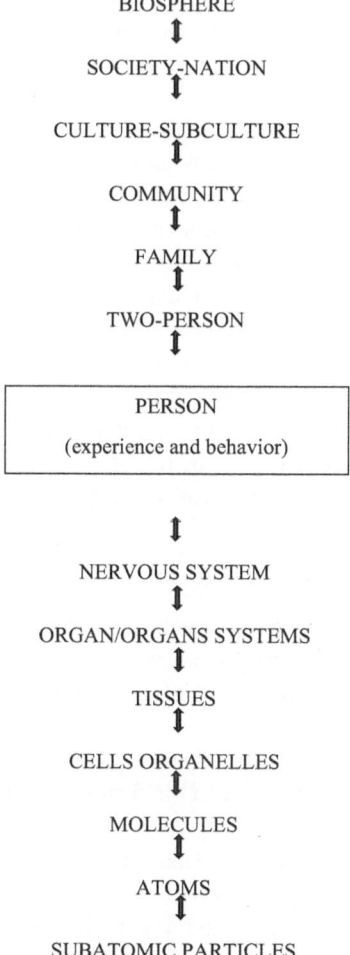

BIOSPHERE
↕
SOCIETY-NATION
↕
CULTURE-SUBCULTURE
↕
COMMUNITY
↕
FAMILY
↕
TWO-PERSON
↕

PERSON
(experience and behavior)

↕
NERVOUS SYSTEM
↕
ORGAN/ORGANS SYSTEMS
↕
TISSUES
↕
CELLS ORGANELLES
↕
MOLECULES
↕
ATOMS
↕
SUBATOMIC PARTICLES

FIGURE 2.1   The original 'Hierarchy of Natural Systems' model of G. L. Engel (1980).

field of medicine. As can be seen, the system 'person' has a box drawn around it, probably signifying there is something special in play here, and Engel notes silently that there are actually two hierarchies in play, one concerning a natural hierarchy and one a social hierarchy.

The clinical part of the article is built around a case of a man suffering from a heart attack, a Mr. Glover. The main idea in Engel's second article is to put the clinical heart failure case into the hierarchy of systems and document that the heart failure is present at every level of the hierarchy. The molecules, cells, tissue, organs, and nervous system are all damaged in different ways; the person is experiencing symptoms and is alarmed; and the social environment at large is engaged and alarmed in several ways, from the spouse over the family to the societal alarming of a rescue team. This multilayered understanding is used through all the phases of the illness, from the first worries over symptoms to an actual cardiac arrest, also involving society's ability to respond to an emergency call, which are depicted in the nine boxes in the hierarchy, with examples of which elements are in play at each stage.

Engel concludes that his case story calls for a doctor with many competencies, as he does in the first article. The doctor would know of the biomedical happenings, be able to relate to the patient's anxiety and that of his wife, know of potential resources in the patient's social environment and in the health systems, and know of the possibility of death. Engel (1980) argues that this model does not impose an impossible demand on the physician: 'The biopsychosocial physician is expected to have a working knowledge of the principles, language, and the basic facts of each relevant discipline; he is not expected to be an expert in all' (p. 543). Engel seems very optimistic about the use of the BPS model: 'A biopsychosocial model is proposed that provides a blueprint for research, a framework for teaching, and a design for acting in the real world of health care,' and pronounces the model has provided 'a suitable framework for scientific study' (p. 543).

2.2 Early critique: What BPS is and isn't

A large variety of critique points have been raised since. Literature reviews of the early critiques have been summarised at least twice (Álvarez et al., 2012; Ghaemi, 2010), and some of the main critique points are historically listed in the following discussion.

The first critiques simply found the model poorly defined and missing causal explanations for the interaction between the factors (Molina, 1984).

> Even when the need of such a model has been extensively described, the model itself and its practical applications had been poorly defined, lacking specially theoretical explanations of the interaction of biological, psychological and social factors in producing medical and psychiatric illness.
>
> *(Molina, 1984, p. 29)*

These points of critique, especially the missing links between the factors, would be repeated several times in the following decades with several attempts to fill in the gaping holes, especially the dichotomy gap between psyche and soma, which would be an ongoing point of critique.

The first very substantial critique was based exactly on that. It was philosophically based and focused on the BPS model version of the body–mind dualism (Goodman, 1991). A. Goodman recapitulated four classic views of psyche–soma relations: 1) psychophysical parallelism, in which mind and brain are different expressions of the same and do not interact (Leibniz); 2) psychophysical dualism, in which mind and brain are two different forms of existence but interact (Descartes); 3) materialism, in which all reality is only physical (Hobbes); 4) Mind–body identity, in which mind and body are two different ways of understanding the same thing (Spinoza).

Goodman found the basic idea of the system's hierarchy based on the principle of *emergence*. On each level (e.g. the cells), there appear properties unique to that level, which can be described to some degree of the properties of the lower-level function, but never completely. When a higher level emerges from a lower (e.g. when organs emerge from cells), the emerged level cannot be predicted or deduced by the components of the lower level. Yet, coherent language and the same logical principles can formulate, describe, and explain the relationships in the level shifts. They are made of the same building blocks, so to speak.

The shifts in the levels of emergence all look the same in the BPS model, but they are not the same, Goodman argues. The shift between the level 'nervous system' and the level 'person' is the very exception (see Figure 2.1). It lacks a conceptual and linguistic bridge, as we have no terms that logically and semantically comprise both mental and neurophysiological phenomena. Goodman concluded that the BPS model is fundamentally dualistic and has not solved the problem it was developed to solve, the holistic view. It requires dualistic thinking.

Some years later, psychiatrist N. McLaren (1998) found that the BPS model is not a model at all, and he argues that the continued use of BPS is unjustified. He stated: 'A scientific model is normally a theory intended to explain a given realm of phenomena or a sort of picture intended to explain a theory by replacing its terms with more perspicuous ones.' He then analyses the clinical case of Mr. Glover and finds no such theory. McLaren proposes that the need for models integrating psyche and soma is so desperate, especially in teaching settings, that nobody has really checked the details of the biopsychosocial model.

Sociologist David Pilgrim (Pilgrim, 2002) defends the model bravely for its 'intellectual resources,' potentially leading to more humanism in psychiatry, but he finds the potential unfolded, as he recognises a powerful return of the biomedical model during the 1990s, which was announced as 'the decade of the brain.' His focus is on the ever-ongoing debate between biomedical and humanistic trends in psychiatry, and he hopes for some kind of rediscovery of the biopsychosocial model, as he sees the holistic striving of the model as a defence for the humanistic side.

In the field of family medicine, the BPS model is genuinely and gratefully praised yet 25 years after its birth (Borrell-Carrió et al., 2004). In a precise and positive tone, Fransesc Borrell-Carrió and colleagues, however, want to update two 'imperfections.' First, they find 'subjective experience not reducible to laws of physiology,' and that it is time to go beyond the mind–body dualism by acknowledging that all knowledge, also scientific knowledge, is socially constructed. They find the categories of 'mind' and 'body' as fragile categories and, to some extent, our own construction, thereby declaring themselves social constructivists. But second, and something essentially new in the critiques, is that they find Engel's concepts of causality limited. The picture of linear cause–effect causality is too simple, as they find real-world causality much more complex and based on circular and structural principles (see Chapter 2.3.2). It is simply not possible to know every cause of a disease, and some causes may come from self-organising structures, which one cannot know anything about.

Psychiatrist Hamid Tavakoli (2009) finds the BPS model to have some pedagogical problems due to the semantic and inherent problems of the model. He also finds the model to dichotomise biology and psychology, and he finds it to reinforce the stigmas associated with mental health by suggesting biology is distinct from psychology. But as something new, he also finds teaching, especially the *social* parts of the model, fundamentally elusive, as the idea of a psychosocial history to be made in the clinic is found too muddy. How can we categorise and differentiate between the sociodemographics of the patient (age, gender, and birthplace), the cultural and religious upbringing, their beliefs, and the economic situation of the patient?

2.2.1   The popular overlapping circles

The best-known image of the BPS model is probably the picture of three overlapping circles with the words bio, psycho, and social appearing on them. As noted above, these images of the model are nowhere to be found in the original articles, nor are they found in the critical articles. The origin of them seems lost in time.

The simple image of the circles might give the viewer an immediate heuristic idea of the holistic ideal of the model, just suggesting that health has different dimensions, as in the WHO definition. The problems with the model become apparent as soon as someone tries to specify the model by putting additional explanatory words into the circles to illustrate what is meant. A Google image search reveals several hundred variations of such circle illustrations. The variations illustrate some of the major problems and the possibilities for genuine misunderstanding of the model. A few anonymous ones are chosen in Figure 2.2.

In one illustration, someone has tried to distinguish what the phenomena in the circles are. As seen, mental health is mysteriously placed under 'biology,' perhaps to give a neuro-psychiatric point of view, but probably more to say that mental illness is a medical speciality. The psycho and social circles are purely non-medical, with

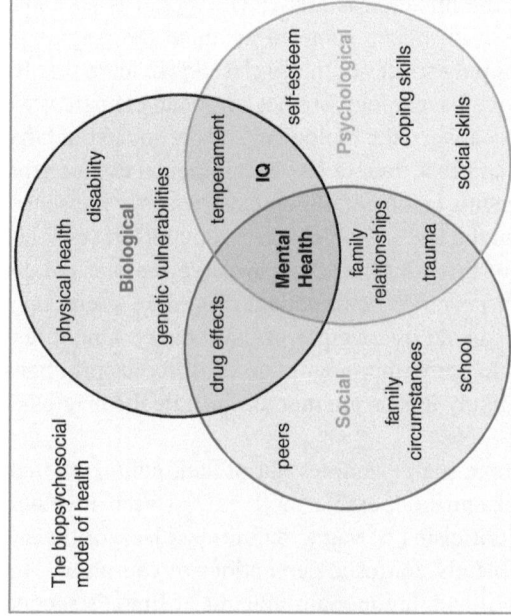

The biopsychosocial model of health

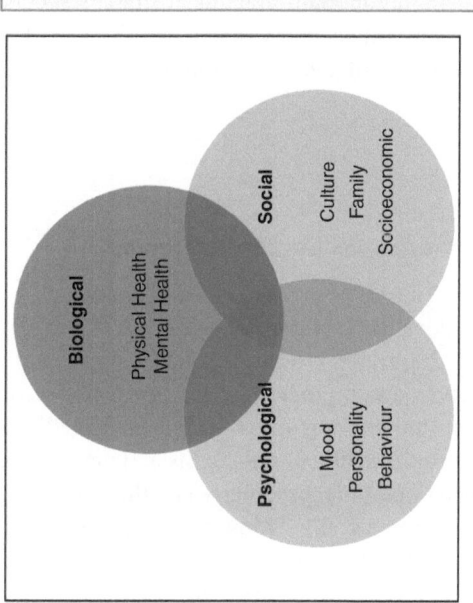

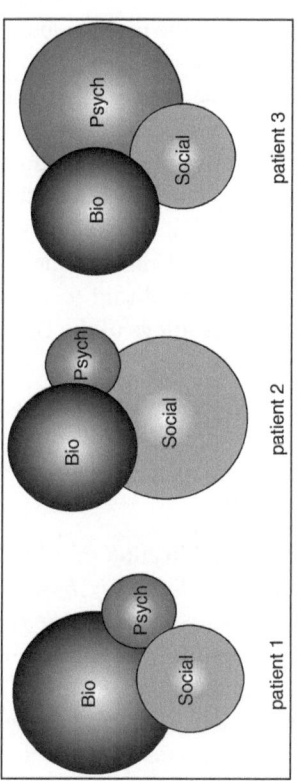

patient 1   patient 2   patient 3

FIGURE 2.2   Anonymous and problematic illustrations of the biopsychosocial model.

psychology described as mood, personality, and behaviour, and social described as culture, family, and socio-economy. There are no examples of phenomena between the circles, and no crossover disciplines involved.

In one other illustration, a clear modification is made: The model is all about mental health, and the model tries to introduce some ideas about the origins of phenomena. It also fills in the overlapping spaces of the circles. So we learn that IQ is something that involves biology and psychology but has no social elements; we learn that drug effects are something between the biological and the social but have no influence on the psychological, and that trauma has no biological component. It might be obvious that these statements taken out of context are nearly nonsense.

The nonsense goes even further in the last example, where thoughts of causality are obviously put into the models of three different patients. We see that patient 1 is somehow more biological than psychological, patient 2 is more social than psychological, and in patient 3, we see an overweight of psychology. One might guess that this is perhaps intended to show the magnitude of different problems presented by the patients, but more likely it is an attempt to illustrate the origins of different illnesses.

Of course, it is totally unfair to take such examples out of their context, which probably has been full of goodwill and honourable motives, but seen together, they might very well illustrate the criticisms of vague definitions, lack of theory, ambiguous nomenclature, and completely confused perceptions of causation. Not to mention that all examples fail to illustrate the main thought of Engel's second article, that all dimensions are always present in every state of a disease. The examples can be said to illustrate well some of the most common and popular misunderstandings of the BPS model.

2.3   Later critique of the BPS model

2.3.1   The missing representation of the first-person perspective and humanism

With the publication of a book by psychiatrist S. Nassir Ghaemi, titled *The Rise and Fall of the Biopsychosocial Model* (2009), the critique reached a significantly higher contextual structure. Ghaemi gives a comprehensive historical review of the origins of the BPS model, based on the striving for eclecticism in medicine and the movement of the 1950s to incorporate different paradigms and maybe also incompatible theories at the same time. At that time, psychiatry had the conflicting psychological theories of behaviourism (I. Pavlov, B F. Skinner) and the theories of psychoanalysis (S. Freud). They were incompatible, and trying to follow both lines of thought resulted in an 'everything goes' attitude, where there were no guiding principles of which sets of thoughts were valid. A movement developed towards seeing the different thought lines as a prioritisation of methods rather than reality. This movement is accredited to psychiatrist Roy Grinker, whom Ghaemi claims to be the real and unrecognised father of the BPS model. Ghaemi also has a very sharp eye for the psychoanalytic and psychosomatic origins of the BPS model, and he suggests that Engel's main contribution is that 'he took the holistic, eclectic, psychosomatic notion of mankind [...] and used it as a weapon to fight what he viewed as the dogmatic biological reductionism of modern medicine' (p. 50).

Ghaemi summarises the historical battles through the times and considers where in the medical fields the model became popular. The model was meant to cover the whole field of medicine, but spokespersons for the model were mainly psychiatrists, more specifically psychiatrists with a psychodynamic orientation. The BPS model historically turned out to be the back door to psychoanalysis and psychosomatics, leaving biology to play a lesser role, Ghaemi concludes.

The resulting main point of Ghaemi's critique is that the BPS model had not changed everyday clinical work for the better but for the worse. The perspective that all levels, the biological, psychological, and social, must be considered in every health task is simply too much for the modern physician, and the result has been *uncritical eclecticism* in the clinic (i.e. 'everything goes'). Ghaemi argues that this eclectic freedom, in which no directions regarding what is essential are given, borders on *conceptual anarchy*. One can favour the 'bio,' the 'psycho,' or the 'social.' The result of this freedom is paradoxical because everyone can continue to enact their personal dogmas, consciously or unconsciously, as there are no guides to prioritisation in the model.

Ghaemi rejects the model entirely. He finds the essential impact of the BPS to be in the battle between the materialistic and the humanistic trends in psychiatry and clinical medicine. But he finds this important battle or dilemma to be better described in the classic works of William Osler (1849–1919). Osler, also called the father of modern medicine, argued for the doctor working as a 'medical humanist' treating living patients and not only diseases.

Humanism (the art of living) and medical biology are not along the same lines as proposed in Engel's hierarchy of systems. They represent entirely different kinds of human knowledge, and according to Osler (and Ghaemi), 'the good doctor' is both medically skilled and humanistic in attitudes and behaviour, seen as two different realities of the patient and two different sets of competencies of the doctor.

Ghaemi represents the perspective of the doctor: the medical view on holistic patient care. The other side, the perspective of the patient, the first-person perspective, the world of the sick person is given voice in a completely other kind of critique. Psychiatrist Allen Dyer at one time became a cancer patient, and in the aftermath, he reflected on his illness and recovery (Dyer, 2011). He is 'thankful for the sophisticated technology such as bone marrow transplant, but it is a grim technology. Without the attentive care of the Duke Staff and the love and support of friends and family, it would have been unbearable' (p. 297). He calls his many thoughts, hopes, and concerns for the illness and his future life 'spiritual,' and he notes that there were no conversations about these important matters with the doctors and the nurses. He does not understand 'spiritual' in any supernatural sense but in a transcendent sense. Probably not aware of any WHO prehistory of the term, he suggests the term 'spiritual' be placed in a bio-psycho-social-spiritual model, which he claims not to be just a sum of the components, but 'a harmonious integration of all the elements of healing' (p. 298). Spirituality is a main key in every healing process, and if it is left out, spirituality is placed in a totally different domain than health and will be handled unprofessionally, he argues.

This is the critique of the missing first person in the BPS model. It was maybe intended in the naming of 'person' in Engel's hierarchy of systems, but it somehow got lost in the further perceptions of the model. There is no actual patient to see anywhere in the overlapping circles illustration, and it is not promising for a model of health that the person who is actually feeling ill is not there.

This is also a main point in the critique from psychiatrists Ana Sabela Álvarez and colleagues (2012). They formulate their work as a 'research critique,' and the critique is based on a systematic literature review of where BPS seems to have been used as a model. They find it employed as a model for combined treatment, a model for reflective processes, and a model in medical education. What they miss is that the model is actually used in clinical applications and in research. They conclude that BPS is a 'perspective and an approach to clinical practice,' and it is *not* 'an empirically verifiable theory, a coherent philosophy, a clinical decision-making tool or a clinical method' (p. 179).

Their main point for not using the BPS as a clinical method is, however, that clinical practice is always a *single-case practice*, and the BPS cannot be a model for this as it completely lacks 'something really inherent in the human being: individuality and subjectivity' (p. 179).

2.3.2   The outdated representation of system theory

Since the times of Engel, general system theory has developed in different ways, and the ideas of causality in living systems have changed a lot. The old idea of 'one germ, one disease' is outdated, and there has been a main shift in the understanding of medical aetiology. That is the main critique by psychiatrist Peter Henningsen in 2015 when he theorised about the BPS in the 21st century. Modern understanding of medical aetiology is about *risk factors*, and these factors can be investigated as biological, psychological, and social on an even basis. We have to work with a 'multilevel empirically based pluralism, which includes the first-person meanings as well' (Henningsen, 2015, p. 363). We need a modernised understanding of the BPS model for such a multilevel explanatory framework.

A proposal for a contemporary rethinking of BPS was published by a group of health psychologists in 2017 (Lehman et al., 2017). They want to improve on the idea of dynamics by applying other models of system theory taken from developmental psychology. Their proposal for modernisation builds on two main ideas. First, they suggested the original threefold division into bio, psycho, and social be formulated as dynamics (i.e. biological, psychological, and social dynamics), putting them as named points on a time circle, as opposed to the vertical model. Second, they suggested a concept of centrality, meaning centrality to health issues. In the middle of the BPS circle, they placed the word 'health.' Potential health factors, such as 'friends,' could be placed near the middle if they were influential to health, or at a distance from the middle if they are not important for individual health. The full illustration was surrounded by 'contextual dynamics,' meaning such things as culture, economy, and environment.

Another positive attempt to update the original BPS model with modernised system theory was published in a small book by Derek Bolton and Grant Gillett (2019), both with backgrounds in neuroscience. They find the original model to be rightly criticised for being vague and mainly used as a 'handwave,' but they want to maintain the BPS model as the general model of health. They want to improve the model by the inclusion of the scientific progress made during the 40 years since the original BPS, and they do so with great insight into modern biology principles, which discards reductionism and physicalism. Their way to make a more (neuro) biological modern model is by reformulating the mechanisms of causation in the BPS hierarchy of systems (Figure 2.1). Simple causation, understood as 'if A then B,' only applies to the physical and chemical worlds, they write. As soon as we

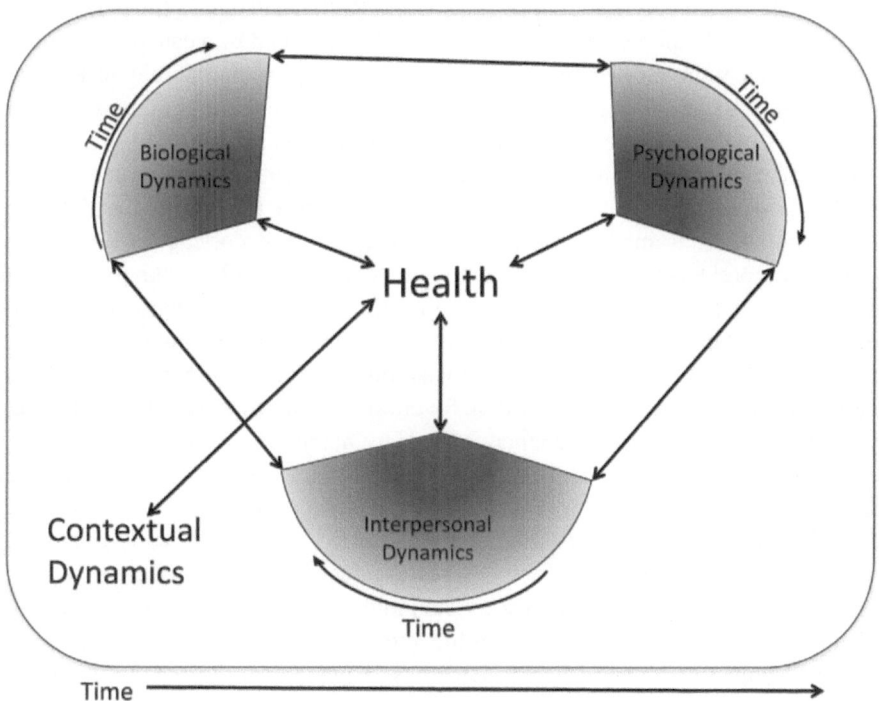

FIGURE 2.3 The 'modernised' BPS model taken from Lehman et al. (2017).

enter the biological world, semantics are involved and interpretations take place, making causations less mechanical: 'A is followed by B in a certain proportion of the observed cases' (p. 24).This creates room for biological errors and for 'multifactorial, interactive causations.'

All living creatures must be seen as complex information systems. This is the basic fact in modern systems theory. There are many kinds of causal pathways in the biopsychosocial systems. 'They can be top-down, bottom-up, and within levels, they can involve regulatory mechanisms, disruptions to regulatory mechanisms, or have nothing to do with regulation, involving energy exchanges only' (Bolton and Gillett, 2019, p. 97). The vertical model of causation is outdated.

As neuroscientists, they also want to get rid of the mind–body split in the BPS model and in our general thinking, and they go so far as to claim a post-dualistic psychology based on the view of the psyche as an information processing agency, which is always embodied. Seen as an information processing agent, the psyche is not different from all general information process principles in biology, they find, and thereby, they do not see any problem with the step from 'nervous systems' to 'person.' They find the only strange step to be that from physics and chemistry into biology, where the rules of causation change from mono- into multi-causation. By this, they argue the biopsychosocial model to be intact when modern systems theory is set as the basic binding principle.

However, on the very last pages of their book, Bolton and Gillett (2019) mention that if anything should be added to the BPS model, it should be a category of ethics and moral dilemmas, somehow acknowledging at least one human dimension that is not fully understood as pure information processing. Their main and important critique lies in the fine knowledge of biological causation principles.

For the explorations in the enigmatic causations between the areas of bio, psycho, and social, a substantial effort to summarise the critique and fill in the missing links is made by Nandini Karunamuni and colleagues (2021). In a very comprehensive way, they map and name the current knowledge of biopsychosocial *pathways*. They argue that the biological, psychological, and social have to be seen as 'distinct systems' which can be conceptually separated, defined, and measured. They then focus on naming a number of modern cross-disciplinary research fields that function as bridges between the distinct systems and possible causal connections. They name, among other disciplines, psychoneuroimmunology, neuroplasticity, social neuroscience, epigenetics, and placebo/nocebo. Thereby, they make a great effort to map out how to make the idea of the BPS system theory plausible, pragmatic, and scientifically related to existing research.

However, they introduce another division in the ideal holistic view on health as they claim health to have two incompatible 'outcomes' to measure: subjective well-being and objective physical health outcomes. A person can be sick not knowing about it and vice versa. By splitting health into two worlds, they are no longer advocates for the unity in health understanding aspired by the BPS model, although they fully acknowledge the crucial importance of the subjective dimension, so much wanted from the earliest critique of the BPS.

Their work called for at least two comment responses, both addressing the understanding of the psychological dimension. An Australian research group (Haslam et al., 2021) takes a social constructivist viewpoint and argues that the Karunamunian BPS-pathways model is too individualistic, overlooking social identities and seeing people in groups. When a young woman leaves home and goes to university, she is not simply the same person in another context; rather, her whole personhood is transformed, as identity is social, it is argued.

The second comment response (R. C. Smith, 2021) points in the opposite direction. Smith finds the individual patient still to be missing in any clinical and scientific use of BPS models. He suggests distinguishing between BPS as a general model (which is not a scientific model but a heuristic tool) and a specific BPS model, which is a clinical one-person application of the model for a given patient. During a patient-centred interview, the clinician will be able to make a biological story, a psychological story, and a social story, and thereby scientifically map BPS factors for the individual case.

A completely new kind of solution to the outdated systems theory in the BPS model is the suggestion of adding technology as a fourth dimension to the model in a 'biopsychosociotechnical model' (Card, 2023). With historical knowledge of both the original model and the critique, author Alan Card adds a comprehensive knowledge of modern systems theories. The BPS systems hierarchy (Figure 2.1) is rightly criticised for being an incomplete model as causations might not be organised in a hierarchy at all, and Card suggests the lens of 'complex adaptive system of systems' (CASoS) – a concept he has borrowed from modern systems theory, (specifically referenced to a theory of engineering tobacco products (!)) but seen as a view on modern health understanding in this way:

> CASoS are adaptive in that the system entities or components can change their behavior, which can result in a change in system structure in response to external stimuli. Additionally, system elements exert directional or bidirectional influences on one another that can change the system structure or behavior. CASoS are also systems-of-systems in that they are comprised of individual but connected systems, each of which is irreducible, and in that the behavior and functionality of the CASoS differ from the sum of the behaviors and functionalities of the individual systems of which it is composed. In a system of systems, not only can each entity be characterized as a system with its own rules and agenda, but the interaction among the systems can cause behavioral or structural modifications within the larger, interconnected CASoS.
>
> *(Brodsky et al., 2011, p. 586)*

This might be seen as a good, contemporary, and comprehensive definition of modern systems theory applied to health causations, and therefore cited here at length.

Card also criticises the BPS for having very little say about improving health, and for being static. He finds the answer to all this to be applying sociotechnical systems to the model in the form of effect modulations of health, such as monitoring devices, robotics, assistive technology, built environment, electronic health record systems, and computer and audiovisual technologies.

Thus, better equipped to manage the complexity of human health, Card still maintains the division of the endpoints, that is,. the health status in two incomparable compartments: physical well-being and psychological well-being. The mind–body split is not integrated, but nicely articulated, as in the work of Karunamuni and colleagues (Karunamuni et al., 2021).

A key medical phenomenon in the BPS discussions has been chronic pain, as it still is a medical 'invisible' entity that cannot be objectified in blood tests or seen in scanning pictures. Furthermore, pain is highly affected by biological, psychological, and social remedies and influences. In the world of clinical physiotherapy, the need for an integrated model is urgent, and also in this field there is disappointment with the BPS and its interpretations. Ben Cormack et al. (2022) describe the BPS model as 'lost in translation' and deeply misinterpreted. They find two different uses of the model present in the clinical field: a 'humanistic' interpretation focusing on persons and therapeutic relationships, and a 'causation' interpretation focused on multiple causations. They find especially the second interpretation misapplied in several ways, by biomedicalisation, by fragmentation, and by 'neuromania' ('overlooking and trivializing non-neural and non-reducible factors beyond the body.' They find a clinical solution to problems by starting with building a relationship with the patient and then openly facing the complexity and uncertainty of the field.

2.4 The general lack of first-person perspectives in medicine

Some of the critiques of the BPS model have origins way back in history and can be rediscovered in many other places in academic writing. This might especially be the case for the problem of the missing first-person perspective in medical practice and rationale. It has been mentioned and problematised at least in the disciplines of medical sociology, psychology, and medicine itself.

The methodological tradition of phenomenology has always doubted the primacy of objective knowledge, knowledge presumably independent of the experience in the human mind. In medical thinking, the question of objective knowledge about the body was raised forcefully by Austrian philosopher Maurice Merleau-Ponty (1908–1961), who emphasised the body as the primary site of the world; all knowledge is placed in the mind, and the mind is *embodied*. We are not able to talk about knowledge independent of the body.

These lines of thought go way back in philosophy and are taken up again and again by philosopher Hans-Georg Gadamer (1900–2002), who thinks specifically about health (Gadamer, 1993). There is always the actual body and the lived body, but it is only the lived body that we can talk about as 'healthy.' There is no meaning in talking of the health of a body that is present, but dead. And further: Health cannot be a concrete experience in itself. It must be defined with other experiences, and Gadamer (1993) goes for the experience of well-being, and 'what is well-being if is not precisely this condition of not noticing, of being unhindered, of being ready for and open to everything?' (p.73). One might find the reflections of both definitions of health in the previous chapter, health as well-being and health as a resource for functioning.

Phenomenology as a method for knowing what is inside another person is the hallmark in the existential philosophical tradition and in the later existential psychology tradition. In this tradition, health will always, first of all, be equal to the experience of being healthy (not feeling ill).

The dilemmas between the physical and the lived body have recently been taken up academically by psychologist Patrick Whitehead in the book *Existential Health Psychology: The Blind-spot in Healthcare* (2019). He argues strongly against the one-eyed objectifying medical tradition, 'where the suffering patient has become irrelevant to medicine' (p. 9). Whitehead has another point problematising the 'medicalization' of everyday life, where health is no longer an absence of medical treatment, but health has become a synonym for medical treatment. There is medical thinking today that does not see the possession of a dog as a part of life itself but rather as 'an anxiety-reducing companion, and gardens are there to dissipate stress' (p. 58), and quality relationships are not seen as the reason to live but an instrument to live. That kind of turning 'the personal into medicine does not *humanize* medicine; it *medicalizes* humanity' (Whitehead, 2019, p. 59, italics in original).

The answer will be the introduction of a new discipline of psychology, existential health psychology, according to Whitehead. It will have the purpose of rehumanising the medical world into the world of living persons with actual problems and concerns, as psychology has become an appendage to the natural sciences, far from the original ideas of the discipline. While medical science is directed to the body, existential health psychologists will be directed at the person, who must overcome new medical issues, Whitehead argues. He has a sharp eye for the medically unexplained syndromes, which are in a particularly difficult situation, caught between the paradigms of modern medical care systems. This will also be a topic later in this book.

3

BACKGROUND FOR A RESTRUCTURED MODEL

3.1 The need for a new model

A comprehensive overview of all the criticisms of the original BPS model does not seem possible as they are too many and too widespread. However, as shown, the criticisms of the model have been substantial, and at least two major points of criticism have been consistently made over the years: the lack of an integrated first-person perspective and a more contemporary concept of illness causality.

Reading through the different critiques, one other common theme stands out. There is a consistent appreciation of the BPS model as representing something very needed. In most of the critical writings, the whole idea of being critical is trying to preserve something that is searched for but not really found in the old BPS model: the perspective of health as a unity, a model of the whole, a holistic account. Almost all the critiques have expressions of the need for a more integrated model of health.

There is a need for an integrated model to:

- stop the spread of medical materialism/reductionism (Engel, 1977)
- pinpoint lack of language for psyche-soma relation (Goodman, 1991)
- unfold the potentials of the holistic model (McLaren, 1998)
- rethink psyche-soma concepts (Borrell-Carrió et al., 2004)
- incorporate humanistic thinking in medicine (Ghaemi, 2010)
- integrate a broad 'spirituality' concept (Dyer, 2011)
- present a first-person perspective (Henningsen, 2015)
- visualise dynamic understandings (Lehman et al., 2017)
- teach a general model of health (Bolton & Gillett, 2019)
- provide integrative (pathways) understandings (Karunamuni et al., 2021)

DOI: 10.4324/9781003502364-4

- minimise misconceptions (Cormack et al., 2022)
- represent modern systems theory (Card, 2023)

This list of needs might also point out cracks and crevices in modern health understanding. There is a need for a modern integrated model of health.

3.1.1 The call from general practice

In clinical work, the lack of holistic thinking is sometimes described as a dilemma or even a conflict between the concerns for society and/or medical guidelines versus concerns for the individual at hand.

1. The scientific perspectives are about what is general, cost-benefit oriented, serving 'the many, but not necessarily the specific.' This perspective can also be named the nomothetic perspective, derived from empirical studies and statistical methods. This perspective is usually formulated as public health policies and often also supported by money with interest, for example by the medical industry.
2. The clinical perspectives are about what is oriented towards a specific individual in a specific context, serving what is good for 'the specific, but not necessarily the most.' This can also be named the deontological perspective, based on insights into the specific person and situation. This perspective is the lived experience in millions of encounters between patients/clients and doctors, nurses, psychologists, social workers, chaplains, and other professionals. These clinicians earn their pay, but there is no actual interest money to promote the perspective in political or scientific respects. This may be the reason why this perspective is much less promoted and easily ignored.

The dilemma and conflict between the two perspectives is well drawn up in a book on contemporary general practice: *Fighting for the Soul of General Practice. The Algorithm Will See You Now* (Shah & Foell, 2023). The authors describe the build-up of tensions between the individual clinician (in this case the GP) and the 'system.'

The motivation for young people to choose an education and career in health or social care may very often be a humanistic wish to make a difference to other people. Making a difference to individual people requires a working relationship with the patient or client. When the system – in the book called 'the algorithm' – takes over in the form of general objectives to be achieved, such as formulas to be filled in, systematic referral of risk groups, enforced advice in particular health behaviours or medication and so forth, the clinicians are in fact reduced to be a 'health machine.' This is far from the original motivation and leads to either low job satisfaction or burnout. The genuine humanistic side of clinical work, the working alliance, is not seen, valued, or paid for by 'the algorithm.'

It is the job of the clinician to balance the two sides of health work in order to do a good job and to maintain job satisfaction, curiosity, and competence, which are the cornerstones in all good clinical work:

> It is therefore an implicit but fundamental part of the job of the primary care clinician to navigate a path of individualised care that is set against the backdrop of standardisation.
>
> *(p. 203)*

> Emotional engagement should be validated instead of being discouraged. Illness narratives do not lead themselves to measurement. Healing is not synonymous with 'sorting and fixing.'
>
> *(p. 216)*

> Algorithm, protocol, and regulation are means to an end [...] and should not have a life on their own.
>
> *(p. 217)*

> A system is needed in which the health workers are permitted to the right thing, even when this means not doing things right.
>
> *(Shah & Foell, 2023, p. 216)*

In the systems and the algorithm, death will always be a failure. But this assumption is just wrong:

> a *good* death should be the measure of the quality of service delivered. However, the factors that support a good death – pastoral care in challenging times, emotional availability and on-going care for the wider family or community – are difficult to measure.
>
> *(Shah & Foell, 2023, p. 12, italics in original)*

The authors also foresee what could be a very important health discussion in the coming years: the growth of artificial intelligence (AI) and its role in modern healthcare. AI is likely to be very powerful and accurate in identifying any kind of risk groups, predicting outcomes of different interventions, and even making accurate diagnoses – in other words, taking over any human involvement and judgement. This can go very far indeed, potentially to the point where the machine makes the decisions, and humans will be reduced to simply carrying out the demands of the machinery. This situation has been, of course, the subject in many good science fiction novels and films, but the medical field may be the first in which it becomes a reality. Humans will then have to define a clear line between the decisions we allow the machine to make about our health and those decisions we define as exclusively human.

3.1.2   Health policies and development

The lack of overview and holistic aspiration in health issues is also present in political processes around health. Health policy, which is often found drowning in the administration of the logistics and technicalities of diverse political decisions, and in the administrative activities, often loses sight of what health is all about. We do not read thoughtful visions of health and happiness in the newspapers; we read about scandals in hospital administration, health staff breakdowns, violation of patients' rights, and sometimes corrupt mismanagement of health finances. It seems like this is what contemporary health is all about: It is about the management and administration of very fixed and frozen concepts of what health used to be, considered in earlier times, with earlier actors reacting to earlier political powers. Political and organisational thinking of health policy is very rarely seen to be visionary into the contemporary health situation, but more an interplay of established, powerful traditions and societies in health management and economic considerations. The 1948 WHO vision of the meaning and purpose of health seems to have simply disappeared.

The issues of health in the wealthy parts of the world are very different from the issues of basic health in the poor parts of the world and in older times, where basic survival has been set as the primary goal. In the rich parts of the world, the purpose of living as long as possible may not be as essential (Ahn et al., 2006) in relation to living a full life, a life of interest and joy, and perhaps not living too long. Dementia follows longevity, and all the mental aspects of health have become more important as seen as dimensions of quality of life. Biology and survival are not the one and only hard facts of health anymore. In all the wealthy parts of the world, we now witness discussions about active euthanasia. The body is functioning, but it is no longer desired that it does so endlessly at any cost. Death may no longer necessarily be a failure.

In the years following Covid-19, there has been a massive increase in the misthriving of young people, obviously a result of social and cultural factors. But somehow, this massive portion of poor health has not really engaged the medical societies or the medical companies; it does not seem to be considered a health problem suited for the existing health system, based on diagnostic categorisations and 'fixing' technologies. The failure of young people to thrive seems to be widely dismissed by modern health policymakers. Engaged in health administration, they may not be well positioned to face the ever-changing health challenges or to maintain a visionary perspective on health.

Health can be seen as a beautiful flower of human civilisation. Human flourishing can be seen as the true wealth, the sign of human richness. But it needs a repeated rethinking of what health is.

3.1.3   The inevitable reductionism and the need for an overview

Another challenge to an integrative model is the way in which medical science develops. 'Divide and conquer' has been the successful motto of the natural sciences for hundreds of years, and it still seems to be the basic principle in biomedical research. The assumption is that a complex problem can be solved by dividing it into smaller, simpler, and thus more tractable agendas. Because complexity is reduced, this strategy is named reductionism. Reductionism has pervaded medical science and has affected the way diseases are diagnosed, treated, and prevented (Ahn et al., 2006).

Reductionism has been a great success. The history of medicine may have its twists and turns and dead ends, some of them grotesque from today's perspective, but all in all, it has been a very positive contribution to mankind. Historically, we can only applaud the reductionist approach in medicine.

Traditionally, we distinguish between scientific and ontological reductionism. Ontological reductionism can be absurd. For instance, if a typed text is reduced to the number of letters in it or to the quality of the paper used, then all the main points of the text will remain hidden. It is otherwise with natural science reductionism: here mankind has made some of its greatest achievements by dividing and conquering complex reality.

In medicine, reductionism has been based on four prominent practices, according to an early analysis of limits to medical reductionism (Ahn et al., 2006):

1. Focus on a singular factor, much like a mechanic who fixes a broken car by locating the defective part. Medical research chases the pathogen, the one cause of illness.
2. Emphasis on homeostasis, illness is defined as a failed homeostatic mechanism, and medicine has the obligation to correct the deviations.
3. Inexact risk modification, the search identification of unidimensional risk factor, the 'one germ, one disease' – thinking
4. Addictive treatments, the assumption that illness problems can be addressed individually and treated side by side, neglecting the complex interplay between diseases and treatments.

Where reductionism explains the biological system by the properties of its constituent parts, systems-oriented approaches will acknowledge that biological systems possess emergent properties that are only possessed by the system as a whole and not by any isolated part of the system (Ahn et al., 2006). The forest cannot be explained by studying the individual trees. This is obvious in clinical work. However, the problem of reductionism is also an increasingly pervasive problem in scientific medicine. Reductionistic medical science has its great advantages concerning 'simple diseases,' for example, urinary tract infections and appendicitis, while it is of much less use for chronic complex diseases such as diabetes and coronary artery disease, as Ahn et al. wrote in 2006.

The problem has only grown since then: complexity is a basic condition in any chronic condition along with the interplay of multiple diseases, which is now the typical disease pattern for most elderly citizens in the rich world. For such conditions, a modern systems perspective must be the integrative part of the understanding. There is a need to make integrative and holistic perspectives easy to get to.

One of the major problems with the tradition of medical reductionism might be that the health system itself seems to be organised by the same basic principle of divide and conquer. The modern health system seems compartmentalised and segregated with ever-growing specialities of excellent expertise, but no overview. Again, this might be fine for simple conditions such as caries control and teeth maintenance, but as soon as things get just a little complex, for example, problematic intolerance to anaesthetics for surgery or a persistent jaw infection, an integrative medical perspective is needed. The same is true for patients suffering from dental phobia, fear of the dentist, being too afraid even to show up, and for patients who want cosmetic but potentially harmful dental adjustments.

Examples of other kinds: Psychotherapy for anxiety may be therapeutically very sophisticated and evidence-based as a stand-alone condition, but anxiety in the context of, for example, ongoing unresolved family problems, workplace problems, a recent attempted rape, or an underlying psychosis, is a desperate need for an overview. What heals one condition might worsen another.

Extensive screening for breast cancer is beneficial in finding early stages of breast cancer. However, there is an ongoing debate about the harm done by extended worrying about cancer and the hell a false positive result brings. Is more harm done than good? (Brodersen et al., 2011).

In intensive care, excellence in pain reduction is often a sought-after skill performed by highly trained experts. For years, the tradition has been that the necessary pain reduction is achieved with such high doses that the patient will die from the medication. The question is whether the person highly trained in pain relief is also a person educated with a good overview of existential issues of life and death and family processes. Probably not.

An integrated overview is a necessity for the many actors in the modern healthcare system. For the system to be coherent and relevant, the many actors need to be aware of each other and the limitations of their own disciplines and paradigms. Awareness of the complexity may be the first step in enabling the actors to talk to each other in a respectful interaction.

3.2 Illness causality and systems theory imagery

The views of medical causality have developed a lot since the days of the biopsychosocial model. Reductionism has led to the idea of mono-causality: one cause for each disease. This idea became seriously undermined with the emergence of public health in the late 1980s, which identified groups of patients at risk of certain diseases (e.g. smoking was identified as a risk factor for lung cancer). The main clash between mono-causality and risk factors is that a risk factor is not a cause in the way that a single agent can be traced as the specific trigger for a disease in an individual. Smoking does not necessarily lead to lung cancer. One might smoke and not get lung cancer, or one might smoke and die from something else long before lung cancer develops. Risk factors are about the health of groups and not of individuals.

Nevertheless, risk factors are the only way to understand medical causation in real life. Complexity is the basis, and systemic thinking is a necessity, as systems from every domain of life are in play in every single case of disease and healing. An example:

If a person *catches a cold* (biological system), this may change his or her ability to *concentrate and remember* (cognitive system), which may push his or her *decision to stay in bed* (personal will system), which may radically reduce the risk of getting *injured in traffic* (public hazards system), but also temporarily reduce his or her *lung function* (physiology system). Low lung function may increase the risk of a *subsequent lung infection* (immunology system). But if *the spouse* (social system) introduces a warm cup of *immune-stimulating herbal tea* (environmental system), the risk for a lung infection might be reduced again.

Now for the question: If this person, in fact, acquires a lung infection, will the cause of illness then be of a biological, cognitive, subjective, public, physiological, social, or environmental nature? The question is meaningless, as all systems will always be at work at any time. There is no single causation to point out. In reality, everything is interconnected, and the best analogy might be a large portion of spaghetti.

In his original article on the biopsychosocial model from 1977, Georg L. Engel came to the same conclusion about all parts at play at the same time, although it was later misinterpreted, as mentioned in Chapter 2.2.1 in this book. However, Engel also contradicted himself by his imagery, which suggested the outdated hierarchy of systems model (Figure 2.1). In the illustration of the model, it seems clear that causation works step by step, either upwards or downwards: Cells organise themselves into organs, and if the cells are sick, they cause the organs to become dysfunctional (upwards causation). Or, if the organ stops functioning, it causes the deterioration of its parts, the cells (downward causation). Within this model, one can, in principle, follow causation step by step by changing the levels of understanding. This way of thinking is not in line with later theories of risk factors and complexity in biological and social systems. The image of the hierarchy of systems misrepresents the modern understanding of causality because it suggests that causation only goes up or down, and because the upward direction is given some priority due to the emergence concept and the naming of a 'hierarchy.'

The model thus conflates two different lines of thinking, that of causation and that of emergence, and the message of the model becomes ambiguous and confusing. The hierarchy of systems model is simply out of date.

Causation in health and illness is not linear (up or down) but *complex*. This means that any element in a complex system can affect any other element, and causation can even be due to self-organising patterns of which we have little or

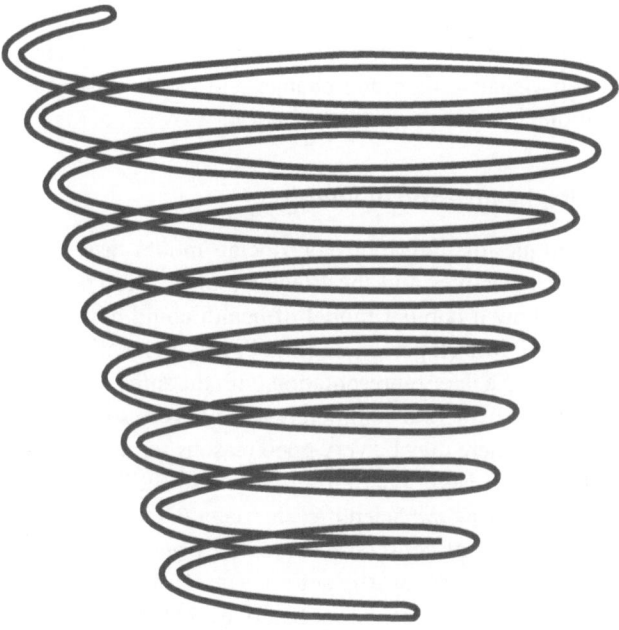

FIGURE 3.1   An up-turning spiral imaging causality in health and illness.

no knowledge, such as homeostasis principles (Marks et al., 2018). In modern systems theory, all parts are interrelated both directly and indirectly. Complexity theory views life as a plurality of interdependent, yet autonomous parts, connected and interacting in a network (Bateson, 2013; Bolton & Gillett, 2019; Capra, 2015; Karunamuni et al., 2021).

A commonly used image of systems theory is usually proposed as a circle with text boxes placed on the periphery and with lines drawn in the centre of the circle connecting the boxes in every possible way. However, this image can be criticised for an association with a static reality, as also mentioned by Bolton and Gillett (2019). A drawn circle does not signal change and dynamics but represents health and illness as a kind of photo, fixed in time and space.

Health and illness are not static; rather, they are constantly moving in dynamic patterns. The health condition of a person is never the same from one day to the next, nor are the person's atoms, cells, organs, social environment experiences, society, and taste of life. The changes are not random but interconnected in patterns that weaken or strengthen each other in the modern understanding of systems theory. All dimensions and systems will always be active in an endless time-spiral movement of causation.

The never-ending exchanges and developments of risks and resources, causes and effects have been proposed to be visualised as an up-turning spiral figure by, among others, Heidelise Als (1982) and Gretty Mirdal (1990). The spiral has a circular motion and will pass through the same causal systems again and again, but it will never position itself at the same point as in the previous round. The up-turning spiral can visualise time and change and can be inserted as imagery for causality in complexity.

3.3 Subjectivity, health, and lifeworlds

A consistent critique of the biopsychosocial model has been the lack of subjectivity: the perspectives and the lifeworld of the sick person. In retrospect, one might wonder how a popular model of health could have existed for so long without any notion of the sick person. In Engel's original work, one might find hints and sentences, but in the later representation with the three overlapping circles, the sick person himself or herself is completely absent. Very strange.

On second thought there may be very good reasons for this situation. The reasons might be that the subject is very hard to place in a scientific way – or what usually exclusively names itself as *the* scientific, the natural sciences. They do not know how to deal with matters of consciousness, so they very often just leave it out, as the consciousness is not there, or it is not relevant. However, a person's subjective experience of illness and health can never be irrelevant to the understanding of health and illness. It is the subjective *experience* of something being wrong that causes the individual to see a doctor; it is the *experience* of well-being that constitutes the WHO 1948 definition of health; it is the *experience of wishes* to be helped that motivates the patient to buy and take medication. It is the experience of suffering and well-being of the body that makes people act in health matters, not the body itself.

3.3.1 The mind–body problem

Certainly, there are problems with maintaining a unified view of the world we live in when we allow the thought of the relation between psyche and soma just a little space. The mind–body problem is unsolved as ever, the gap between the first- and third-person perspectives. It is an enigma, a mystery.

Try this little experiment: Bend your index finger and stretch it again – maybe three times. While you are doing this, try to think about how you are actually doing it. How do you make your finger move? You do not command it to do it; you just want it to, and then it bends; it obeys your will and desire. But what does your will consist of? Can you feel it in any particular place? No? The will is usually not even conscious, but in this case your will reacted to something read in a book – not printed letters or atoms, but content, suggestions that are themselves without atoms.

It is the same with memories and dreams – they are not made of atoms, so what are they made of? The 'thing' that is amused by humour and makes your body smile and laugh, where is it situated? The body, the matter, is smiling in reaction to something which is itself matterless.

Your body is almost always complying with you. It moves to the right or left according to your matterless purpose, and during your lifetime, it has complied all the way with one's choice of professional education. In this way, the body is the servant of the mind; mind is over matter.

On the other hand, your psyche is a slave to your body and brain. When one drinks alcohol, the psyche changes. The abilities to think and concentrate are given by the brain, the emotions arise and exist in the body. When you fall asleep, your body has commanded a mandatory requirement and then switched off the main switch to the conscious experience. And the final proof: When the body dies, the subjective and consciousness are no longer present in the shared world, if at all. The matter is over mind.

Mind over matter and matter over mind, both statements are 100% true. The epistemological mystery may be as old as mankind itself and can be traced far back in the history of philosophy, in written form back to Buddha (c. 450 BCE) and Plato (c. 300 BCE). In the Western context, it became a clear medical problem when the church slowly loosened its reluctance towards systematic dissection. Public dissection was allowed and popular in 'anatomy theatres' during the sixteen hundreds, and corpses for this purpose were often criminals and misdoers delivered by prisons. The mind–body enigma then became public: Where in the dead body was the criminal seeded? The depraved nature and the criminal misdoer were nowhere to be found in the body (Koenig, 2000; Park, 1994; Porter, 2003). Philosopher René Descartes was also a curious dissector and came to the conclusion that there were two kinds of matter in this world: *res extensa*, the substance of the extended, and *res cogitans*, the substance of thinking and unextended things. This viewpoint is often referred to as radical dualism.

Later, philosophy and epistemology gave consideration to these matters again and again in different combinations and relations, as for example mentioned in Chapter 2.2. A way of making an overview of the many varieties of positions is seen in Table 3.1.

It is an independent point that even though the different views are almost like beliefs that you can subscribe to or not, in everyday life we all operate with many ideas about the relationship, depending on what we are talking about or which clinical domain we are working with. You can simultaneously recognise a neuropsychiatric starting point, for example, but also find it meaningful to work with narrative medicine, which has a completely different assumption about the psyche-soma relationship. Apparently, this is not a big practical problem. But for a model of health and illness, it needs to be properly represented. The psyche-soma problem cannot be approached without a deep respect for the tradition that has covered it for centuries. There is no quick fix.

Although neuroscience has made great progress and has been transformed in the most recent decades, the essential problem remains untouched. Brain mapping can tell us which areas are involved in specific processes, but it cannot tell what persons

TABLE 3.1 Different views on the relationship between psyche and soma

NAME	Mechanical materialism	Dialectic materialism	Objective idealism	Subjective idealism	Solipsism
One or two dimensions	Monism	Dualism	Dualism	Dualism	Monism
Psyche-soma-relationship	The material, objective, is the only thing that exists	The objective is the primary that creates the subjective	Two independent, interlocked processes	Subjectivity is primary, creating and shaping the objective	The subject is the only thing we can know exists
View on consciousness	Consciousness does not exist independently; it is purely epiphenomenal	Consciousness is an epi-function of the nervous system that it acts back on	Consciousness has an independent existence parallel with the objective	Consciousness gives existence to the objective	The objective world does not exist in itself
Examples of advocates	Thomas Hobbes Ludwig Feuerbach	Karl Marx Aleksej Leontiev	Gottfried Leibniz Carl G. Jung	Edmund Husserl Stanislav Groff	George Berkeley
Examples of implicit thinking in the clinic	"Device failure models" Neuropsychology	Neuropsychiatry Health psychology	Psychosomatics Psychoimmunology	Narrative medicine Experience-centred psychotherapy	Existential conversation Dreamwork

are thinking, what they are dreaming about, or what their opinions are. Cells can organise as tissues and organs, but they are still made of the same building blocks, molecules. We do not know what makes up the consciousness, but we know it is there, our fundamental knowledge of being alive. The radio mechanic may know everything about electrical circuits, and he can potentially follow every atom in every wire, but even with this sophisticated knowledge, the radio mechanic cannot know anything about the radio programme broadcast. The programme does not 'emerge' from the radio itself; it has a world and rules of its own. This is the mind–body problem in a nutshell.

We can certainly wish for and search for a unified understanding, or just to get closer to it, but we still do not have a unified understanding, not even the building blocks for it. We have to be pragmatic towards our lack of bridges over the gap between mind and body. We have to acknowledge each in its respective dimension. There is nothing wrong with a pragmatic pluralism (Pigliucci, 2008). It tries to describe the world; it does not try to explain the true nature of it.

3.3.2   Dimensions of human reality

The basic dichotomy is also a key point in epistemology, the theory of knowledge. There are also two dimensions of knowledge that are not in line, but do not function without each other: the knowledge of the objective world and the knowledge of the values of it.

Good examples of what is at play here can be found in philosophy and psychology from the early 1900s. Philosopher William James spoke with a little odd wording of the distinction between an existential judgement (a judgement about 'constitution, origin, and history') and a proposition of value (a judgement about 'importance, meaning, or significance') (James, 1902). Danish philosopher Harald Høffding spoke in more intuitive understandable terms about the *category of reality* and the *category of value* (Høffding, 1916). The thoughts are the same, and Høffding probably took them from James. In any case, their main point is that we cannot deduce from one category to the other. James gives the Bible as an example: One can count the letters in it, determine the number of writers, and describe the content of it in detail (categories of fact); but from that one will never be able to conclude that this might be the most important book in world history (category of value). And vice versa: Knowing the Bible as maybe the most important book in history (category of value), one is not able to deduce anything of what is in it (category of fact). There are two sides to the coin; we are not able to see both sides at the same time, and the images on the sides of the coin are usually very different. A pragmatic acknowledgement of the two worlds of knowledge does not solve the problem, but it makes it clear and visible.

The big question is what we as humans are capable of knowing about. We are not really able to know anything about infinity because we basically cannot grasp what it is. Nor do we really know what space is, other than theoretically. As Augustine wondered: If no one asks me what time is, I know what it is. If I want to explain it to the one who asks, I do not know. Human knowledge seems to follow the human life-space, the human world, the world as we see it.

We tend to group our knowledge in dimensions, which are dimensions in the experienced human lifeworld, dimensions we are usually not aware of. Our Western academic tradition has identified four such dimensions of knowledge. Again, William James will be the first advocate for classifying our possibilities of knowledge into four categories (James, 1890). He writes phenomenologically about the Self that it constitutes itself into two classes with a pair in each, which he named the *material Self*, the *social Self*, the *spiritual Self*, and the *pure Ego*. Also here, the chosen wording might lead modern understanding a little astray, but in James' explanations of the chosen terms, we find these meanings: 1) The material Self is the body. 2) The social self is how others see us. 3) The spiritual self is 'the psychic faculties and dispositions' (cognitive apparatus and personality traits). 4) The pure Ego is the ego that is felt, the self that experiences life, while in itself is difficult to detect or to think about, it loses itself in 'some bodily process, for the most part taking place within the head' (vol. 1, p. 300). The idea of a division is clear, although the naming of the dimensions is perhaps very old-fashioned and the scope of thinking about the four dimensions is not fully unfolded.

This basic division of four dimensions is found again in a very unfolded, modern, much more elaborated and comprehensive version in the works of Ken Wilber, especially the book *A Brief Theory of Everything* (2007). Wilber employs a broad scope in his attempt to make a theory of life in the cosmos, and his main idea is the division of reality into two basic axes of the world, the one called interior

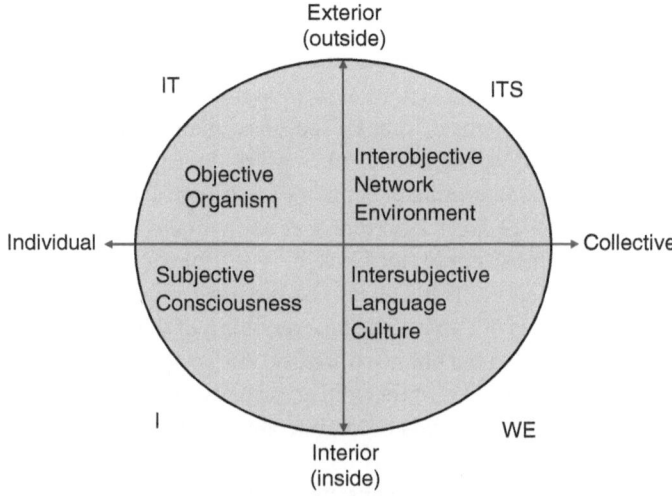

FIGURE 3.2 A circumplex and adapted model of the dimensions suggested by Ken Wilber (2007).

and exterior, the other called individual and collective. Placed as a cross, this basic idea leaves four fields of existence, which represent the dimensions of *subjective, objective, intersubjective, and inter-objective.* In Figure 3.2 the axes of Wilber are put as opposites in a circumplex model (two dimensions placed as a cross), and some of Wilber's explanatory naming of the dimensions are included. (The content is Wilber's, but the endpoints of the dimensions have switched around from Wilber's original model due to adaption to later representation of models.) Wilber's model later had several applications and is now named 'the quadrant model' (Fernandes-Osterhold, 2021; Ferreira, 2018).

To bring the thoughts of division into four parts back close to the concepts of health, we might look into the model by psychologist Emmy van Deurzen-Smith (Van Deurzen & Arnold-Baker, 2005). She builds on the works of philosopher Ludwig Binswanger (1963), and she reflects on how human life can be experienced in different dimensions (see Box 3.1). She announces four 'life dimensions' in which life can be experienced, named *physical, social, personal, and spiritual.* Looking more closely, it may be noticed that small differences separate the models of Wilber and Van Deurzen besides the obvious naming differences of the dimensions. The word 'culture' is placed in two different dimensions.

BOX 3.1   THE FOUR DIMENSIONS OF EXISTENCE ACCORDING TO VAN DEURZEN (2005).

- Physical (*umwelt* – 'things'), including body and health
- Social (*mitwelt*, 'others'), including relationships and culture
- Personal (*eigenwelt*, 'self'), including character and dispositions
- Spiritual (*überwelt*, 'life'), including meaning, will, good, and evil

---

The common feature between these models is the striking agreement on the quadrant structure. I guess more examples could be drawn in.

In relation to the biopsychosocial model, which names three dimensions, the fourth dimension occurs by a split of the 'psyche' into two. One psycho dimension comprises intersubjective psychological phenomena that are observable, conditioning the psychic life (habits, dispositions, learning, language), which could also be summarised as a cognitive/behavioural dimension, the 'known.' The second psycho dimension is the subjective dimension of experience, which is not observable from the outside, but private until expressed to others (i.e. the experience of being alive as a continuity, experiences and sensations of the body, experience of meaning, happiness, well-being). It is the 'I' looking through the eyes, the stream of consciousness, the 'knower.'

4

THE FOUR-DIMENSIONAL MODEL OF HEALTH AND ILLNESS

The division of human reality into four dimensions appears to be robust in historical, philosophical, and epistemological terms. However, the theories mentioned above do not share a uniform common naming of the four dimensions, and they do not share much of the associated paraphrasing that further describes the dimensions, but they do share the basic ideas. If a new four-dimensional model of health and illness is to be proposed as a better-suited heuristic model than the BPS, space is needed for adjustments, adaption, and contextualisation of the associated content of the four dimensions.

The new model proposed here will have a visual representation as shown in Figure 4.1.

Within this model, the basic four-dimensional structure is kept as in the logic of the quadrant (subject vs. object and private vs. public). The model has five up-going spirals, symbolising causality, one small in each dimension and one larger encompassing all four dimensions. The spirals swirl in the dimensional matrix.

The suggestion is that human health can be conceptualised in four dimensions, all of which can be considered separately as healthy or not healthy, functional or dysfunctional. The dimensions are all *interrelated*, but because we do not have concepts or language across the dimensions, they are also *distinct*. Although theoretically derived, the four dimensions can also be perceived as very pragmatic in that they reflect, to some extent, the current organisation of modern healthcare in the Western world.

4.1 Characteristics of the four dimensions one by one

The four dimensions are, in short, considered in turn below. The coverage follows elementary common expressions of the dimensions in a systematic way but is not intended to be linked to any particular health discipline or profession.

DOI: 10.4324/9781003502364-5

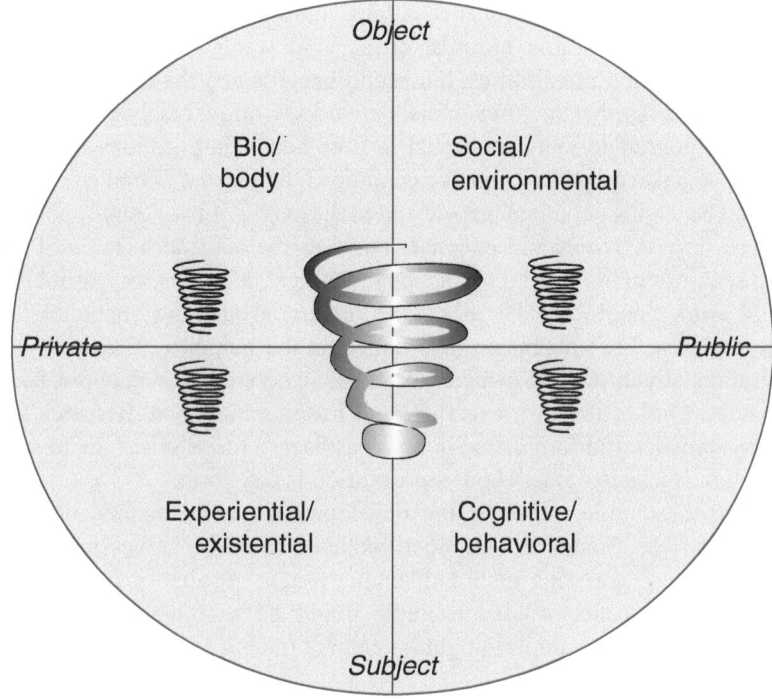

FIGURE 4.1   The four-dimensional model for health and illness.

The first dimension, 'bio/body' (top left), represents the natural science, biological perspective. Bio encompasses health in relation to the private, material body and comprises the body as an object.

Bio stands for all processes of health, illness, and healing processes that can be described positively in biological and medical terms. Bio links the concrete individual to basic biological functions, including the principles of regulation and homeostasis in the body (e.g. digestion, immune system, hormones).

Research is usually done within natural science framing and is usually represented by disciplines such as biology and biomedical sciences.

An example of a bio/body routine in the clinic might be taking a blood sample and analysing it for specific antibodies. Examples of treatment modalities can be pharmacology and surgery. A cancer-related example of bio-dimension might be a tumour, which is described and diagnosed as the uncontrolled growth of cancer cells. An example of a bio-perspective in an epidemic disease might be that the disease is seen as a virus and with a vaccine that needs to be developed.

The second dimension, 'social/environmental' (top right), represents health and illness in relation to the environment, surroundings, and structures shared with others, describing our common external reality.

The environmental concerns health and illness in relation to the objectifiable surroundings, the material environment and its resources such as the availability of clean water and food, a clean breathing atmosphere, the absence of toxins, but also things like traffic hazards, crime, and war. The social encompasses social structures and possibilities; the health benefits and the risks of groups and society, such as family structures, social networks, workplaces, health politics, and the sociodemographic facts connected to this; health implications of education, economy, social segregation, housing conditions; and so on. Social/environmental health can be positive components viewed as the availability of things, possibilities of leisure time activities and exercise, but also the societal hazards of adverse events, such as environmental toxins, poor political decisions, or humiliating and stressful work conditions. There can be functional and dysfunctional families and workplaces. The dimension also concerns the health system itself seen as organisation, structures, and availability of health services, for example, hospitals, pharmacies, clinics, health prevention, and health economics. Research is often based on statistics and formulated in terms as hazard ratios or risk factors. Health intervention is usually understood as prevention in any form.

A clinical example might be the development and communication of new nutritional advice. Standard 'treatment' methods could be prevention initiatives, but also political decisions such as planning a new hospital or improving work environments. A cancer-related example might be a stop-smoking campaign. During an epidemic, examples might be contact tracing and infection monitoring of an infectious disease.

The third dimension, 'cognitive/behavioural' (bottom right), represents health and illness in the context of the broad cognitive science, that is, those dimensions of the psychological world that relate to our shared experienced reality. It is the intersubjective perspective, the part of a person that is known or can be known by others. It is the intersubjective, objectifiable perspective of the inner individual, often based on what has been *learned*: the language spoken, common knowledge, observable behaviour, cognition, and emotions, including the typical characteristics of relationships with family, friends, colleagues, and networks. It is the person seen as trained and formed by adaptation to the context. Cognitive/behavioural concerns the aspects of health and illness that are linked to the traits and behaviours of the person, for example, the person's habits, dispositions, tendencies, and social adaptations, and the person's developed intelligence, cognitive style, talents, and personality in its exchange with social reality and groups. It is linked to biology in that it represents the psychological expression of the capacities of brain and body functions in cognition and behaviour. Cognitive/behavioural includes all observable moods, modes, and problems. Mental health and psychiatric illness are included in this dimension when recognisable by others.

Research in the field is usually performed with a variety of methods, including observational, experimental, quantitative, and qualitative methodology.

Clinical examples of illnesses in this dimension could be the diagnosis and treatment of depression or stress when these are treated with cognitive psychotherapy or behavioral regulation as the main principles. In the case of cancer, an example might be a patient's observable tendency to self-isolate during the illness. In the case of an epidemic, the example might be the individual's actual change in behaviour in order to avoid infection, for example, keeping a social distance.

The fourth dimension, 'existential/experiential' (bottom left), represents the *humanistic* perspective on health and illness. It is the dimension of personal experiences, personal orientations, and their possible expressions. First of all, it is the first-person perspective, the 'I' that looks out of the eyes, the 'I' that experiences suffering and well-being. It includes the experienced body, the bodily sensations, perceptions and pains. The experienced body is constantly scanned for sensations and feelings, and one can feel well or sick. It also includes any personal health decisions made on the basis of bodily experience, for example, the decision to seek a doctor or not.

The existential/experiential dimension encompasses the individual's personal evaluations, orientations, reflections, and choices. It is the truly subjective dimension grounded in the experience of being alive and participating in the world, of being existent. The existential/experiential dimension comprises the inner experience, where the 'one who thinks' makes considerations in relation to the world, valuing it. It comprises health and illness with concepts as meaning, hope, will, purpose, life satisfaction, the joy of life, and all genuine choices in life, as well as the opposites: meaninglessness, hopelessness, agony, suffering, lack of engagement, and living without direction. Existential/experiential also encompasses dreaming, fantasies, and the perception of art and storytelling. Existential health is not about biological life, living space, or cognitive abilities but about living a life valued as worth living. The field covers the sources of meaning in life, personal values, ethics and basic assumptions, world views, religion, and the choices and actions based on them. It is the experienced quality of the lived life. It is the dimension of 'a good life' as well as well-being and suffering.

Thoughts and possible acceptance of personal death also belong here, which make death positively relevant as a health topic.

Humanistic sciences are involved with disciplines like anthropology, philosophy, theology, and humanistic-oriented psychology, disciplines that hold the subjective experienced world as a reality. It can also be present in the medical profession when the humanistic sides of the discipline are considered. Research in this field is usually rooted in the phenomenological tradition (qualitative research) but can also include other methodologies such as imaging and interpretation, hermeneutics.

Examples from the clinic: Some feel sick but are well in laboratory tests; others feel well but have abnormal lab tests. Some feel they are well connected to the body and are very careful in keeping up good health; others are not cautious about this and want quick technical fixes. Some can accept illness; others cannot. Some engage; others capitulate during illness. Some experience loneliness even when surrounded by others. Some die from meaninglessness and sorrow. Some choose to commit suicide.

Treatment elements based on this dimension are numerous, but an example could be the commitment to a good quality of contact during counselling about a possible abortion. It is the humanistic side of 'the good doctor' and can potentially be every health professional who is able to hear and talk with patients about

TABLE 4.1 Keywords from the four dimensions are placed schematically

Dimension	Bio/body	Social/ environmental	Cognitive/ behavioral	Existential/ experiential
Type of science	Natural science	Social science	Behavioral science	Humanistic science
Area	The private, material body	Environments and structures	Relations, dispositions, language	Orientations, choices
Disciplines	Biology, medicine	Public health	Psychiatry, psychology	Humanistics, psychology
Example clinic	Blood analysis for antibodies	Nutritional advice	Stress	Feeling ill
Example treatment	Pharmacology and surgery	Water quality check	Psychotherapy	Choice of abortion
Example cancer	Tumour understood at cell level	Stop-smoking campaign	Depression	Will to live
Example epidemic	Developing vaccines against a virus	Contact tracing	Keeping social distance	Fear of infecting others

existential issues, a good life, health orientations, and health choices. There is a growing need for attention to this due to the still increasing number of chronic diseases, ethical dilemmas and choices, and the enormous complexity inherent in modern health systems.

An example in the context of cancer might be to remain connected in hope during the disease process. An example during an epidemic could be the individual's conscience and caution not to infect others and the personal ethics behind self-isolation.

4.2 Limitations and abilities of the four-dimensional model

The four-dimensional model represents a simplification of reality like any model. The model is suggested as *a heuristic model for understanding health and illness in modern society, not as a model of the world.*

The most important thing about the model might be that it recognises that all four fields are health-related and fully present at all times; none can be left out, but one or another can be focused in a specific health context.

Some aspects of human reality will not fit anywhere in the model, and others will be essentially present in multiple fields. 'Culture' is an example of such a multilayered concept and is not named anywhere specific in the model. Culture is not a 'thing' or a 'process'; it is everywhere. Culture is a concept extremely hard to define as it is all-pervading (Hatala, 2012). Culture could very well be understood as best represented in the social/environment dimension as suggested in some models mentioned earlier, as culture can be understood basically as our human-made surroundings and artefacts. However, culture is also fully present in biology as the body develops and takes shape under certain cultural conditions such as food traditions and fashions. Culture is indeed cognitive, as it is the specific language learned, the concepts, expressions, focus points, and so forth. And culture is fully existential as it provides frames for our world views, ethics, and religion. In fact, it has been convincingly proposed that culture should also be understood in a 2 x 2 factorial design, very much like the four dimensions suggested here (Carriere, 2014).

Some health concepts very hard to place could be 'lifestyle' or 'compliance.'

On the practical level, the boundaries between the dimensions may be set mainly by language, research, self-understanding, and practical handling of the different scopes in the dimensions. The four-dimensional model suggests that an image of holistic health should be held when talking specifically about health in one of the four dimensions: physical health, social health, mental health, and existential health. Each dimension has possibilities for unfolding and for development in linguistic and scientific concepts and expressions.

One of the most interesting things about modern health may be the borders between the dimensions, especially when it comes to the understanding of causations between them. There are opportunities here for new and integrative research. As mentioned above, the work by Nandini Karunamuni et al. (2021) maps cross-disciplinary borderlands with research areas like psychoimmunology, stress/

HPA axis, placebo, stigmatisation, life events research, and the like. These are promising and upcoming research fields. But, as Karunamuni et al. also point out, these areas have to deal with the challenges of integrating two or more languages and scientific understandings.

Thinking about the borders of modes of understanding is always exciting, but not anything new to the four-dimensional model. What are the boundaries between living and dead matter? The boundaries of inner and outer, the private and the public? When a person thinks a thought, it is internal and private; the moment it is put down on paper and read by someone else, it is external and public, but still also fully internal and private. Another border very difficult to get totally sharp is the border between the cognitive and the experiential. We have a clear image of many of the incommensurable differences but not of the exact separating line, just like the other boundaries.

A model is always a balance between what is captured for the ease of understanding and what is left out for the ease of understanding. There is no end to such thoughts about health and illness, but thoughts may 'harden' in a fruitful way for a period of time.

On one hand, the model aims to emphasise the wholeness of human life and health, and on the other hand, it aims to fully respect and not mix up different dimensions of health as represented in the many health disciplines. The spirals illustrate that the biological, psychological, social, and existential are constantly changing and exchange conditions for themselves and each other, which function as chains of causation in the complex system.

The four-dimensional model for health and illness is proposed as a name, as the term 'biopsychosocial-existential' seems unmanageable. The term 'biopsychosocial' may still function as the best wording, but maybe with some notice that the model is rethought.

Health is always the health of both *something* and *somebody*; it is both objective and subjective. The proposed model does not bridge the gap between mind and body, nor does the model make any attempt to do so. It acknowledges that the gap exists out of respect for our different modes of thinking, and the model makes it visible. This viewpoint could be called *pragmatic dualism*, pragmatic for the greater course of a holistic view of health.

The image of complex interactions within and between different systems replaces the principle of mono-causality, whether of physical, psychological, social, or existential nature. Treatment and interventions to meet illness are usually built on very few links of causation, of which we have some understanding and some ability to change in a conscious way. However, successful treatment of causal links in one health dimension does not mean that the illness only exists and is real in that dimension.

The four-dimensional model is presented for a more comprehensive understanding of health topics in clinical work, organisations, health policy, and especially within health education, such as medicine, psychology, public health, nursing, physiotherapy, social work, occupational therapy, and chaplaincy.

PART II
What is existential health?

5
EXPLORATIONS IN EXISTENTIAL HEALTH

What is new in this book is the inclusion of existential health. It is therefore appropriate to attempt to develop and unfold this concept further.

The word 'existential' is by no means new; it is part of our cultural history in countless ways, and it continues to evolve in new directions and meanings. In the following, some of the key ideas in both classic and modern understandings will be presented along with existing definitions and models of the concepts.

5.1 What makes a topic existential?

5.1.1 Existential philosophy

Existential thoughts – thoughts about what human existence is really about – have been around for as long as we have known ourselves as humans. In palaeontology, one of the theories of what distinguishes humans from apes is the evidence of burials with burial gifts around 100,000 years ago. When a gift is given to the dead, it is a sign of belief in some kind of afterlife and, thereby, some ideas of what reality is and the nature and role of being human in that reality. They are thoughts of existence.

Existential thoughts have historically been a major part of religious myths, stories, and dogmas, telling about life's strains and quarrels, the nature of suffering, and the individual's role in the bigger picture, often promising a final righteousness and a blissful ending stage of existence and pointing at a right way of living.

In Christianity, the inner life had at least two main streams possible to flow. For the sincere, there was a possibility to live an inner life of contemplation, prayer, and meditation, striving for inner peace and reconciliation with the saviour. For the

DOI: 10.4324/9781003502364-7

ordinary, inner life was told to be the story of sin, shame, guilt, forgiveness, and punishment, which are the major stories.

Existential thoughts have also been the main content of many philosophies, but the name of existential philosophy is of quite a new date. It is mainly concerned with the purely subjective perspective, a life seen from within, the experience of living, and also ideas about the right way to live the inner life. The name existential philosophy is associated with a group of loosely connected thinkers who wrote in a little over a hundred years of European cultural history (Cooper, 2003).

Existential philosophy is said to have its roots in the works of Søren Kierkegaard. One main reflection for him was 'the self relating to itself,' meaning that we are able to relate to our own inner lives and that we are existing in the world; we are self-reflective. But from there on, a large bouquet of different ways of thinking emerges. Some are deeply religious (e.g. Kierkegaard, Buber, and Marcel), others hardcore atheists and averse to religion (e.g. Sartre, Nietzsche, and Camus).

Throughout its disjointed and contrasting history, some key concepts associated with existential philosophy have stood the test of time. A rather common speculation is the relationship between *essence and existence* – which is the question of what exists in reality. For example, does a table or a book exist outside of our perception of them? In themselves, they are just a collection of atoms, and as specific objects, they are meaningless to, for example, an ant. For an ant, the book and the table would be 'obstacles.' With this point of view, it is our human perspective on the world that determines how the world is perceived, not how the world really is. Our perception determines what is called reality.

Deeply linked to existential philosophy is the *phenomenological method* (described by Edmund Husserl). It is the gateway to know something about the inner life of another person and to explore another person's perspective. The method later became known as the basic interview stance in qualitative research, and it is often also considered the basic approach in existential psychotherapy.

According to Ernesto Spinelli (2005), the phenomenological method can be described in three steps:

1. Rule of epoché: Putting aside our initial prejudices and preconceptions about things in order to suspend our expectations and assumptions.
2. Rule of description: Describe, do not explain. Stay with the lived experiences as they are.
3. Rule of horizontalisation: Avoid initial hierarchies of significance and treat each item of description as having equal value or significance

Another characteristic of the existential tradition is the determination that *each individual is unique*. There is only one of each of us. There is only one who experiences being alive and living this particular life, and this only one may share the world with others but is still uniquely alone (e.g. Irvin D. Yalom). This is a highly individualistic perspective.

On the other hand, we are only someone because *we are with-others*. We cannot exist alone in a void; we are basically always with others; we are human beings in the power of others (e.g. Buber). This is inherently a strongly collectivist perspective.

Existence is also fundamentally seen as *a process* – a stream of being – and existence can never become a thing or object in itself. Existence is dynamic, a flux, an ongoing event, a path, to use some of the terms that have emerged in the tradition.

It is also a core assumption of existential philosophy that in existence there is always a *free choice*. Here, existential philosophy often stands in stark contrast to other philosophies and world views, perhaps especially the more scientific ones that emphasise human determination by biological processes, unconscious patterns, and societal conditions. The paradox between the two views is a core philosophical question as well as the body–mind question. Existential philosophy will claim that, whatever the circumstances, human beings will always have the free will to relate to circumstances in a chosen way.

Existence is seen as something stretched between the past and the future, *an eternal now* that is ever-present, anticipates the future, and has just disappeared into the past.

There is the question of finitude – our inevitable *death and the awareness of it*. Here, again, we find irreconcilable views represented; for some, death is a characteristic of limited existence; for others, death consciousness is a way into deeper forms of existence, perhaps most clearly in the form of religious fulfilment.

We exist in the world, not outside of it. We do not know existence outside of our being in it. For many philosophers of existence, *we are the body* because our experience of being is completely tied to the body. Our experience of being is a 'psychosomatic whole.' We are *embodied*, many in the tradition argue, while others disagree.

Life is full of *dilemmas* and *paradoxes*, and living freely between them is seen as the ideal life. This is the more ideological thought about *authentic life* as the only life to strive for and represents some very normative considerations of life that are also part of existential philosophy.

Anxiety – the Kierkegaardian *angst* – is an expression of existence; it is claimed. Angst is a result of our free will. When we choose, we can also choose wrongly and thus be responsible for our own misfortune. We can regret and experience *existential guilt*. But if we live in awareness of our freedom, life can be lived with passion, creativity, and vitality, where existential anxiety and guilt are companions. An authentic life is not without suffering; suffering can be the very expression of an authentic life. However, we can also choose to live less strongly, inauthentic, to tone life down and end up in 'the common indifferent averageness' where we are 'deadened, domesticated, tranquilised and alienated from ourselves' (Guignon, 2002).

There have certainly also been strong critical voices against existential philosophy. Mick Cooper (2003) mentions four main criticisms where things do not add up:

• The philosophy is anti-essentialist, yet describes certain characteristics of human existence.
• There are existentialists who advocate finding one's own innermost truth individually, and there are existentialists who advocate that it is only through encounter with the Other that life is given meaning.
• Existential philosophy is essentially amoral in the emphasis on human freedom, self-creation of values, and the lack of any absolutes.
• Existential philosophy is over-morbid with its focus on despair, anxiety, guilt, and death-awareness. (pp. 20–31)

Existential philosophy is not unison and cannot be done justice in a small space, but it is characteristic that its most significant proponents wrote their main works more than 50 years ago. Although the philosophy itself has not been significantly renewed since then, the core existential concepts seem to resonate more and more, but now often in contexts other than philosophy.

That will be the topic in the following discussion.

5.1.2 New understandings of 'existential'

In recent academic literature, the meaning of the word 'existential' seems to have shifted with a number of new, common associations. It seems to have evolved into a much broader concept that is by no means better defined, but which also seems far removed from the categorisations and dogmatics of traditional existential philosophy.

A recent article empirically examines the meaning of the word 'existential' among normal Danes (Hvidt et al., 2021). Using factor analysis, the authors find three common meanings of the word in a secular population:

1. Essentials to 'a good life' – with associations such as family, health, security, identity, belonging, gratefulness, and quality of life
2. Spirituality/religion – with associations such as believing in something bigger, why God has created me, greater purpose, meaning of life, and ideas of life after death
3. Existential thinking – with associations such as existentialism, life's big questions, deep thoughts, and to exist

The term 'existential' itself does not seem to be alien to the common language, but the meanings go in several directions, and only one meaning refers to existential philosophy, while the other two refer to a secular understanding (existential seen as 'a good life') and to a spiritual/religious understanding (higher meaning of life).

For years, there has been a huge amount of scientific research into the relationships between religion, spirituality, and health (see later). In this literature, spiritual and religious are not the same thing, but there are no clear dividing lines between the two concepts. It has been heavily debated: Which is the larger concept? Does religion include spirituality, or does spirituality include religion? (Moreira-Almeida & Koenig, 2006).

The fuzziness of definitions of 'religion' may be well known, and the concept of spirituality seems even more elusive (see Chapter 1). An empirical study in 2012 asked ordinary Danes about the meaning of the word 'spirituality' and used factor analysis comprising meaning units (la Cour et al., 2012). The authors found as many as six different meanings that had little to do with each other. However, the first factor was again associated with well-being and 'the good life,' while the second factor revolved around New Age ideology (astrology and healing etc).

In the field of medicine, there has been widespread scepticism towards using the term 'spirituality' in the health system, perhaps especially in Scandinavia. In 2006, Swedish oncologist Pär Salander (2006) criticised the use of the term 'spirituality' in oncology journals. He felt that the word 'existential' was a perfect substitute, 'who needs the concept of spirituality,' and he believed that advocates of spirituality did not like the term because it is related to existential philosophy's denial of God.

An attempt to tidy up this conceptual mess in medical research was made in an article by the present author and a colleague back in 2010 (la Cour & Hvidt, 2010). The main idea was to review the definitions of the terms religious, spiritual, and secular orientations, using the word 'existential' as an umbrella term: all three world views cover different *existential orientations*. The article reviewed known definitions from the academic literature: secular existential orientation, spiritual existential orientation, and religious existential orientation. This was done with respect to each dimension, including 1) the words used to describe it (cognitions), 2) the practices connected to it, 3) and the potential personal importance to the individual.

In this way, 'existential' was used as the main term for possible life orientations that are not bound to any philosophical tradition.

5.2 Existential health definitions

5.2.1 Existential health as meaning-making

The first known attempt to define existential health that the author is aware of came from Valerie DeMarinis (2008) in Sweden. She focused on the word 'existential' as an underlying process of making sense of the world, building a reasonably coherent world view, and the word 'health' as related to whether or not this process was successful. DeMarinis linked existential health primarily to the public health dimension, asking whether young people's difficulty in finding a coherent world view had implications for mental health and social instability:

> The existential dimension is focused on the individual's understanding of existentiality and the way meaning is created. This dimension includes worldview conception, life approach, decision-making structure, way of relating, and way of understanding.
>
> *(DeMarinis, 2008, p. 60)*

Her initial notions of existential health are thus connected to the public or collective practice of meaning-making activities in the same way as religion and spirituality has meaning-making qualities. She sees such practices as cultural expressions threatened by secularisation, postmodernism, and immigration in the postmodern world. We need to be aware of a decline in existential health and be able to prevent it with public existential health initiatives, planning for 'existential societal well-being,' she argues.

A few years later, Swedish theologian Cecilia Melder (2012) followed this line of understanding, leaning on DeMarinis:

> A postmodern situation, which presents the individual with too many choices, can lead to mental dysfunction if a person is unable to make a choice, unable to make meaning, affecting their ability to make life decisions.
>
> *(Melder, 2012, p. 243)*

Melder defines existential health as 'a person's ability to create and maintain a functional meaning-meaning system' and asks how this dimension relates to health dimensions such as 'self-rated health' and 'quality of life.' Over the years, Melder and colleagues have worked hard to develop a model of public health, culminating in the proposal of the 'rainbow model of determinants of public health' (Dyar et al., 2022). This model includes determinant effects on health by social support, trust, meaning in life, and hope. Their later work is closely related to the faith and interfaith aspects of existential health and the WHO questionnaire for spiritual, religious, and personal beliefs (WHOQOL-SRPB) (Melder, 2022).

5.2.2   Existential health as pure subjectivity

Theologian Ola Sigurdson, who has a background in Barthian theology, completely disagrees with the considerations of DeMarinis and Melder (Sigurdson, 2016). He argues against letting existential health be a separate category of health, and he argues that existential health – what he understands as the experience of being alive – will be superior to all other understandings of health. Existential health is vertical; other forms of health are horizontal. Citing the main point of the work of Gadamer, he states that 'health is not a condition one introspectively feels in oneself. Rather it is a condition of being involved, of being in the world' (Gadamer, 1996, p. 113). Sigurdson defines existential health as 'a reflexive feature of human subjectivity in relation to health,' and by that existential health is and will always be *unmeasurable.* In a later work, he defines existential health as 'the art of suffering.' He argues that we achieve good existential health through the process of 'learning how to suffer' (Sigurdson, 2019).

Suffering as the basis for existential health seems to be a very ideological but often heard claim based on a very narrow part of reality. It is true, of course, that one does not gain much experience of life and possible wisdom without adversity and crisis, which are often painful. The first serious love break-up during puberty is rightly called suffering, and most people mature from it, and it makes possible a later adult, meaningful relationship having learnt the basic lessons of love life. Suffering is certainly a core concept in existential health, but suffering is by no means the main road. Most suffering is utterly meaningless. Believe me, I have worked for many years as a clinical psychologist at a clinic for chronic pain. There is little wisdom and growth to be gained from ongoing chronic illness and pain. It is just suffering with no inner meaning or message in the same way that starvation catastrophes and the bombing of civilians are. There is absolutely no need to embellish that.

In his recent book *Existential Health: The Blind-Spot in Healthcare* (2019), psychologist Patrick Whitehead also takes the position of defining existential health as subjectivity. He has a strong point when he argues that patient suffering is, in principle, 'irrelevant to medicine' (p. 9). He gives historical reasons for this: when medicine became an empirical science, it focused very much on the *observable*, which further led to the idea that the observable became synonymous with *real.* He notes that this objectification of illness in medicine has led to a dichotomy in modern medicine: Products of medicine and the medical providers are good, while any kind of suffering is bad. Our lives are becoming 'medicalised' – a term he borrows and revives from philosopher and social critic Ivan Illich (1975).

A patient does not *feel* a broken leg or cancer, which may have enormous consequences for the future life and existence. But neither the *feel* of the illness nor the consequences for the lived life are central in medicine, where only the objectified categories of illness are considered *real.* Modern medicine cannot validate the patient's suffering (Illich, 1975, p. 28).

In defining health, Whitehead draws heavily on the philosopher H. G. Gadamer. Gadamer defines health as well-being (as WHO 1048), but he adds something very important: 'What is well-being if it is not precisely this condition of not noticing, of being unhindered, of being ready for and open to everything?' (Gadamer, 1996, p. 73). One could paraphrase that health defined in this way might be close to the WHO 1984 idea of health as a resource.

Whitehead (2019) clearly sees existential health as the subjective and suffering side of any illness. From there, Whitehead takes an unexpected turn, calling for a new field of *practice* in medical care, a practice capable of taking human suffering seriously. He calls this field 'Existential Health Psychology' and argues for a new health profession akin to hospital chaplaincy, but without religious presuppositions (p. 63). He calls for the new health professionals to be humanistic and holistic in their scope, practising 'existentialism at the hospital' (p. 68).

Narrative medicine and existential phenomenology are seen as the main remedies in this new field of practice, both regarded as methods or guidelines for conversations that focus on the life story of which illness is a part, and on the concrete bodily experiences throughout the course of the illness.

Being very practical, Whitehead (2019) gives four steps at the end of the book, as an 'antidote for medicalization' (p. 105):

1. Treat the how, not the what (exchange the body with the person)
2. Illness, not disease (the feel of the illness)
3. Treat not the disease that has the person, but the person who is ill (care more for the person than for features of the disease)
4. Caring for an Other (make the relation a human–human interaction)

5.2.3 Existential health as reflecting the 'existential givens'

From early in the tradition, some existentialists tried to identify essential existential characteristics. Martin Heidegger spoke about the main 'existentials,' and he listed them as these: Caring, Understanding, Being-with, Being towards death, and Mood.

The idea of a limited number of 'existentials' – also called 'givens' or 'ultimate concerns' by later existentialists – can be reduced to an even simpler collection according to the American psychotherapist Irvin Yalom (1980). Yalom himself identifies only four existential givens:

1. the inevitability of death for each of us and for those we love
2. the freedom to make our lives as we will
3. our ultimate aloneness
4. the absence of any obvious meaning or sense to life

As seen, these are quite different from Heidegger's earlier list, but Yalom argues that he can simplify the existential essentials to exactly these four givens because they are of particular relevance for *psychotherapy*, which is the field of expertise in which Yalom has written and rightly earned his fame. He sees *mental health as a reconciliation of the four givens* in a person's life. Although embedded in the existential tradition, Yalom is quite different in the style of conversation he uses, having been trained in psychoanalytic methods. He does not favour the phenomenological principles, which are otherwise claimed to be the main road to the understanding of another subject, and he is very thoughtful about being personally open in the therapeutic process, thereby questioning the value of authenticity that other existentialists hold high.

Modern existential psychotherapy might be found in the British School of Existential Analysis with names like Spinelli and Van Deurzen-Smith, both mentioned earlier in this book. They are ardent advocates – one might call them fundamentalists – of the phenomenological method. They do not speak of 'givens' but of 'three principles for existential phenomenology,' which they find are: Relatedness, Uncertainty, and Anxiety (Spinelli, 2014). Again, a goal of psychotherapy (and thereby also a sign of existential health) is to reflect and reconsider these principles.

The Norwegian psychologist and psychotherapist Per-Einar Binder has recently written a concentrated and readable review of the concept of existential health: 'Suffering a Healthy Life – On the Existential Dimension of Health' (Binder, 2022). He reflects on both the 'existential' and the 'health' concepts, and he tries to combine the existential as subjective with the simplicity of the 'givens.' However, he finds Yalom's four givens somehow one-dimensional and wants to phrase them together with their opposites, forming polarities. He also finds that in the context of health, Yalom's four givens are simply missing out on the body, and he basically adds the bodily experience, making his list of existential givens look like this:

1. Awareness of death, and insight into the way it enriches our being, for example, to invite making life choices in line with what we experience to be most important in life
2. Creation of meaning, collectively and individually through language and culture, engaging us with other human beings and goal-related tasks. Meaninglessness and lack of purpose is always a latent threat
3. Connectedness, life is fundamentally relational and our lives deeply connected to other people, but we are also isolated, as parts of us are out of reach from others
4. Freedom, we are fundamentally free and responsible, but at the same time also limited by our habits, our un-awareness, social structures, and power limits
5. Body experience, feeling ourselves, relating to what is going on in our inner selves as embodied being-in-the-world with both strength and vulnerability

At the end of his paper Binder (2022) concludes:

We might become healthier through our existential struggles; meaning is essential for a healthy life. But at the deepest level, we do not face our existential challenges to become healthy. We struggle with them because purpose, meaning, and existential concerns are of the highest value for our lives. In a highly medicalized society, we need to reinvent our language for these existential struggles, and the suffering that always accompanies them.

If a concept of 'existential health' can make us more aware of the fact that the existential concerns are always part of both health and illness, it is worth developing. (p. 6)

5.2.4 Existential health contextually and empirically defined

The previous attempts to define existential health have mostly represented a 'top-down' strategy, where the thinkers determine what the words are about. It is top-down in the sense that one or more thinkers, philosophers, theologians, and psychologists have tried to work out how the words 'existence' and 'health' gave meaning to them in some kind of systematic way, giving suggestions for categories and distinctions.

Another strategy for investigating what is in a word is the bottom-up strategy, which does not make many assumptions in advance, but looks at how words are used and understood in the world around us, our context. This has to be done in the specific context of interest.

The bottom-up methodology has been the strategy of the research group around Swedish Peter Strang. For more than two decades, this group has added insights to existential topics such as physical pain and existence (Strang, 1997), existential loneliness (Sand & Strang, 2006), and extreme death anxiety (Strang, 2014), simply by asking people in the field about their experience with these topics.

A good example of this method at work is the study of the concept of existential pain (Strang et al., 2004). The research group sent questionnaires to 173 hospital chaplains, 115 palliative care physicians, and 113 pain specialists, asking them to answer the question: 'How do you define the concept of existential pain?' The results showed that existential pain was mostly used as a metaphor for suffering, but with some interesting differences in context: Chaplains were more likely to emphasise guilt issues, palliative care physicians – actually working with dying people – were more likely to emphasise separation and annihilation, while pain specialists were more likely to emphasise that life itself is painful.

A very recent Swedish study used the same method to analyse existential loneliness and meaning-in-life in nursing home residents. They interviewed residents themselves (Larsson et al., 2024). They combined the qualitative data with theoretical and empirical work relating the concepts of existential loneliness (defined as the inability to bridge the gaps that exist or may arise between ourselves and others) and meaning-in-life (defined as a buffer for holistic well-being when stressors arise), and they found that both concepts are important and basically not met in the everyday life in the nursing home. They find three themes that further describe the landscape: Being seen, Trust in life, and Looking forward, themes that could also function as gateways for interventions and conversations on existential issues.

Very important for further exploration of the concept of existential health itself is the extensive literature review of the word 'existential' in the context of

Scandinavian healthcare journals from 1984 to 2020 (Nygaard et al., 2022). The authors find that the term is increasingly used, but rarely defined, and there *appears to be no consensus on the meaning of the term.*

Marianne Rodriguez Nygaard et al. (2022) categorise the use of the term 'existential' in the 138 articles included in the review into five overarching ways of usage. Existential meant:

1. *Suffering and re-orientation.* The relationship between suffering and a better state of being. Suffering is often referred to as chronic illness, physical pain, loneliness, and depression. Hope and re-orientation were associated with situations described as finding relief, comfort, new understandings, and other resources.
2. *Meaning and meaninglessness.* This theme was often linked to a lack of meaning (e.g. in depression and burnout) and to the process of meaning-making and the relationship with meaninglessness. It was also closely associated with themes such as existential suffering, loneliness, and existential resources.

These two themes were found to focus on dynamics in people's lives, while the next three themes had other anchors.

3. *Existential philosophy in relation to health.* This was based on the theoretical framework of existential/humanistic philosophy and psychology, and the names mentioned in the article are Laing, Rogers, May, and Yalom. It focuses on the holistic being-in-the-world that applies to everyone, healthy or sick. Special attention is drawn to the 'given' of existential isolation (loneliness), which seems to be well represented by associations such as hopelessness, despair, anxiety, powerlessness, vulnerability, and longing.
4. *Existential questions as an approach to care.* In the nursing specialty of existential and spiritual care, care is often described as one's being able to listen to and support a patient's existential questions, questions such as What is meaning in my life? or What would happen if I took my own life? In this way, existential represents a field of practice, of being aware of existential questions as a caring professional.
5. *Usage and demarcation of existential, spiritual, and religious concepts.* Inconsistencies and interchangeability between the terms existential, spiritual, and religious were found in the literature. It is not clear which term best encompasses the others. Looking at the research traditions from which the concepts were described, a pattern emerged that the word 'spirituality' was mainly used in nursing research as an umbrella term for the concept of existential. Existential philosophy mainly used the word 'existential' without any notion of the others, while the tradition of the psychology of religion used the word 'existential' as an umbrella for secular, spiritual, and religious domains.

In the discussion section of their article, Nygaard et al. (2022) consider which tradition and wording might best serve the purpose in health contexts. They argue that the word 'existential' has a long tradition as a neutral and better category for an overarching concept. It might be understood as an impartial term, encompassing the secular realm without 'transcendent undertones.' Increasingly combined with health perspectives, it can be seen as the concept 'filling the gap in a society that wants alternatives to transcendent resources' (p. 15).

After all their reading, discussing, and categorising, Nygaard et al. (2022) venture to make their own definition of existential in the context of health, seeking a broad and consensus-like approach by naming selected 'givens' that make the most sense in relation to health and naming three world view orientation systems.

Their definition is this:

> The term 'existential' in the context of health embraces the basic conditions of being human, the dynamics of suffering and reorientation, meaning and meaninglessness and, finally, secular, spiritual and religious worldviews.
>
> *(Nygaard et al., 2022, p. 18)*

With this definition, we are brought much closer to a manageable corpus of existential health.

5.2.5   Existential health associations

In an attempt to gather common understandings and associations of the term 'existential health,' I have been asking for associations of the term 'existential health' for a number of years. This has led to the collection of some very basic data, which has not been published elsewhere.

5.2.5.1   Method for data collection

Over a period of about 5 years, the same question was asked every time I, the author, spoke at a lecture, seminar, conference meeting, or the like with health professionals such as physicians, psychologists, chaplains, nurses and a few times students of the disciplines. The question was: 'What do you associate with the concept of existential health?' and participants were asked for topics, matters, reflections, supplements, and critiques.

Intensive notes were taken and transcribed each time as *data collection*, resulting in a still-growing Word document of the associated terms. In the course of time, 20–25 groups of 5–35 people have contributed and discussed topics within the field, totalling approximately 350 persons; no exact count of participants was made.

5.2.5.2   *Data handling*

The Word document grew and reached its maximum with about 500 different words and concepts. (Some random examples of the raw data: guilt in illness, curiosity, balance, attitudes to the body, feeling and emotion – what is their role?, health choices, lack of orthodoxy, acceptance of suffering, what is natural death? etc).

The next step in data handling was a process of *grouping words*, similar to the process in qualitative data work, giving each concept one or two nodes and then *grouping the nodes*. (For example, grouping 'lack of orthodoxy' with 'flexibility in world views'). After that, the next step was to eliminate words that covered similar meanings and *concentrate* the data sheet into fewer elements.

On a continuous timeline, some more theoretical elements were added, trying to relate the terms and grouping them into ideas and concepts that could be refound in contemporary health literature, philosophy, psychology, or social science literature. At a certain point in time, a 'List of elements in existential health' was presented at a conference in Groningen, Holland, in 2023, containing this list of 14 concept groupings comprising 35 terms and concepts:

- Belonging, Connectedness
- Sense of significance
- Purpose, Destiny
- Coherence, Inner homeostasis
- Autonomy, Internal locus of control, Freedom of choice
- Self-confidence, Guilt/consciousness
- First-person perspective
- Experienced continuity, Experience of body, Personal history
- Existential well-being, Quality of life, The joy of life (happiness)
- Meaning in life
- Identity feeling, Self-image
- Hope/Optimism, Life thirst/existential engagement, Curiosity, Existential loneliness/boredom, Flexibility in world views
- Attitudes to the body, Nature and the relation to it, Life orientations, Beliefs
- Death consciousness, Acceptance of death, Suffering, Acceptance of suffering

This data-driven list still looked messy and was out of focus, but it represented work in progress. What was then added was a theoretically and empirically based reconsideration of the structure of the concepts and groupings, leading to the suggestion of a map of the terrain of existential health, formulated in the next chapter.

6

MAPPING THE TERRAIN OF EXISTENTIAL HEALTH

Before we take any preliminary steps towards a more comprehensive drawing of the elements in existential health, let us consider some of the characteristics we might look for in a description of the content.

We want the drawing to be broad and inclusive, not excluding anyone interested in the field, not to please anyone in particular, but broad enough to be understood by all health professionals, including doctors with a biomedical orientation, health administrators, researchers, and health politicians. Ideally, it should bring together both empirical bottom-up perspectives and theoretical top-down perspectives in order to reach both theoretical or ideological health promotion projects and pragmatic health research.

It should be grounded in the real world in such a way that it is possible to identify domains, areas of practice, and empirical findings that are clearly relevant for existential health.

It is important not to make a final definition the ideal, not even for a consensus understanding, but to provide a picture worthy of further reflection and development. If we look at physical, psychological, and social health as we did in a previous chapter, none of them has a fixed definition. But they do have an area on the map of health that more or less exclusively bears their name. Why should we have different or more rigorous requirements for the area of existential health? If we can define a ground or a landscape on which houses of many different kinds can be built and considered a city, we have come a long way. The map is not the landscape, but it is a very practical place to orient yourself.

DOI: 10.4324/9781003502364-8

6.1   Categories of components in existential health

The empirical information of what is associated with the existential may have been covered to some extent in the previous section. It is clear that the existential dimension must consist of many elements or groups, just as the physical dimension has groups of elements, for example, internal organs, skin, or immune system, all of which can be evaluated as healthy or non-healthy. But before we consider health, we need to consider the elements themselves.

In choosing the elements, their names, and groupings together, it seems important for future use and development that the wording and theoretical thinking be consistent with concepts already known in psychology, philosophy, and health research. This will make it possible to place what is already known about the elements and their relationship on a firmer footing, perhaps even to suggest relationships between the elements.

The interesting part from here would be to see whether any ordering or ranking of the elements in the existential field is possible. To do this, we could go back to the basic four-dimensional model and think of a new direction within it, namely the direction across the dimensions, in this case, from the bottom left corner and to the centre.

It seems fundamental that the element in the bottom left-hand corner will be the pure subjectivity experience as such – that which cannot be shared with others (absolutely private) and is inner (not reducible to elements of the outer). To draw the full line across, one could speculate what would be the extreme opposite: the

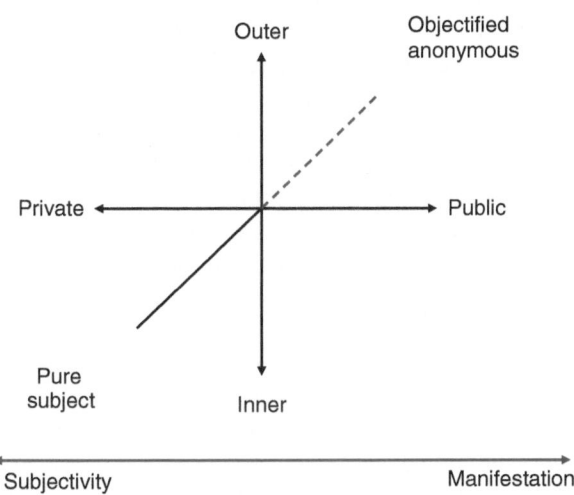

FIGURE 6.1   The cross-line between the subject experience and the anonymous objectified person.

dimension of a human being fully seen from the outside and all public, with no subjectivity recognised. It would be the human seen in human statistics: the anonymous person described as a citizen, as a voter, as a member of the labour force, or as the count of military soldiers. It is the rational, objectified individual who plays a role in cold political rationale.

In the existential field, which elements could be said to be placed on the cross-line line from the pure subjective experience and towards a slightly more outer and public space, that is towards being slightly more visible to others, but still private and inner? The second layer, in my view, will be the systems of life orientations, the things we believe in and trust without much grounding. The third layer will be the still a little more visible or public accessible layer of the qualities that are the results of the orientations. It is the orientations that we actually live as persons with more or less success; it is the orientation parts of our lives that are describable as characteristics of us as individuals. The fourth layer is very close to the outer and public world and can be described as the expressions of the experience of living, the orientation systems, and the qualities, perhaps as others can see them in obvious personal expressions such as political commitments or religious affiliation, maybe even as personality characteristics of the individual.

From this way of thinking, an order of the elements in existential life can emerge as follows. The direction and sequence is to look at things from the pure inside and follow things on the way to the outside.

Experience of living. This is the layer closest to being purely subject, the first-person non-reducible element and category. A prominent claim of existential thought is that the subject cannot be fully shared with others. The experience of being alive in a life context, of having a consciousness, is unique. The subject is indeed embodied and continuously engaged in a moment-to-moment evaluation of the body on a sensory basis, scanning for well-being and suffering, joy and pain, and anything in between. The subject gets also fully psycho-embodied and socio-embodied, during infant development, and thereby also becomes aware of immediate states of suffering and well-being as psychological and sociological identity.

This continuous scanning, listening to, and evaluating perceptions, thoughts, feelings, and bodily sensations results in the sense of self, the feeling of 'I' as an identity. This sense of identity is even given a name. The subject looking out of the eyes is named and exists as a somebody, recognisable in the mirror. The relationship between the subjective awareness and the somebody can be called the self-image.

Part of the constant subjective evaluation of being in the world, which cannot be fully shared, is the sense of meaning in life, or in some circumstances, the sense of crisis of meaning in life. Is life worth living? Not as a theoretical question, but as a pure and lived scanning of the life experience. Without knowing anything about it, almost everyone judges most of the time that it is more worthwhile to be alive than not to be alive. This is the sense that life has some meaning in itself.

Somehow the subject also contains some inner and individual dynamics. The preferences and consequences of these inner life dynamics are without any external witnesses and often not even conscious to the thinking subject itself. It is the life of dreams, visions, and longings, experienced while asleep, fully awake, or in states in between. This kind of inner life dynamics can be horrifying, like suffering in nightmares; but it can also turn out to be guiding lines in one's personal life, like a calling or a longing for certain surroundings or special tasks and obligations to be pursued. They can be thought-provoking or affirmed, like in art perception of any kind. They can change life orientations in revolutionary ways in visions and in trances as near-death experiences. If we want to formulate it more poetically, it is the soul.

Without the non-reducible category of the subject, its well-being, and suffering, it is meaningless to talk about health of any kind. If it is not there, we are dead.

Life orientations. These are the subjective, evaluative, and meaning-making processes that result in daily life orientations and a possible coherent world view. They are the subjective attitudes, the basic assumptions about what life is and what gives it meaning and value. The orientation systems shape our individual faith and belief in things, and they identify the individual sources of meaning in life. Such life orientations may be fixed and unchangeable for some, while others may have more floating and changing orientations. The orientations also include the internal attitudes towards our body; some people are very careful with it and keep it fit and healthy, some worship it as it was the purpose of living, and some regard the body as an instrument or an object, usable and repairable like a car, until it stops working. Orientations are about the internal relationships with the external world, with nature and our place in it; some feel a strong coherence with nature, others see it as an enemy of civilisation, and some see it preliminarily as an opportunity for personal gain. All orientations can be of an individualistic or a self-transcending nature and they have possibilities to evolve during a lifetime.

Existential qualities. These are evolved results of the existential orientation system, still subjective, but somehow also partly visible to others in words and behaviour. The qualities are also characteristics of inner well-being, or the opposite, and they can be formulated positively (with well-being) or negatively (without well-being), for example, as living a meaningful life versus living a life with no meaning. Living a life with meaning could be the main term here, as qualities such as purpose in life, sense of significance, and sense of coherence and belonging can be seen as elements in meaningful living, but somewhat more visible to others in the sense that it can be talked about and recognised in another person, but still not shared.

Another word for the same thing might be quality of life, which is also not fully visible but, in some respects, can be made an object for further investigation.

Being existentially engaged or living with existential indifference are inner qualities, almost characteristics of a person, as are basic curiosity, life thirst, and hope, as well as the opposite qualities.

Seen from the inside, qualities such as self-confidence can be the effect of a well-functioning life-orientation system, as well as the opposite, guilt and shame. Like other personal qualities, named in personal psychology, such as inner homeostasis, autonomy, and inner locus of control (ability to choose), they can all be seen as results of inner orientations, but as we approach existential layers closer to the external and collective world, the dependence and shaping of such qualities by outer circumstances play a greater role for them, as the qualities can be recognised and talked about.

Existential expressions. With the existential expressions we are close to elements partly or maybe already measurable in some form. We are able to see, hear, and recognise expressions of happiness or grief in another person, although the experience of it is subjective. Obviously, there are also expressed world views in the form of political attitudes and statements, and in faith and belief organised in the collective world. Some expressions can be called life philosophy, such as expressions of viewpoints and the existential 'givens,' for example, death consciousness.

Subjective decisions about one's own life are also often openly expressed, for example, the choice of living space, education and work area, spouse, the decision to have children, and so on. Many life decisions will become objective facts, shared in common, but still based on individual, subjective choices.

Some existential expressions can be seen as expressions of individual qualities, such as, for example, generosity, which is also named as a personality trait when viewed from the outside. Some personality traits can be developed based on life choices and existential orientation. For example, it is possible to develop an accepting attitude towards suffering and death for ourselves, as well as in our fellow beings and nature. Attitudes of neglect or denial are also possible, and everything in between. We are now in an area that is very close to ordinary psychology and very much mixed up with it in the sense that we are able to talk about these traits and describe them, and we have some ideas about measuring some of them on scales and correlating the elements to other things.

Art expressions might also be closely related to personality traits but are also often an existential expression in itself.

If the proposed structure of the layers and groupings of existential elements were graphically represented, like a primitive map, it might look like Table 6.1.

The theoretical framework of meaning in life in the present book mainly follows the conceptualisations of Tatjana Schnell (2021), who classifies meaning in life into different categories of unfolding and action. These categories are here named as three and placed in different component groups on the existential map (Table 6.1)

- *Sense of meaning*, which is considered as the very subjective and immediate sense and evaluation of life as meaningful;

TABLE 6.1 The existential map: A structure of groupings of existential components

EXPERIENCE OF LIVING	LIFE ORIENTATIONS	EXISTENTIAL QUALITIES	EXISTENTIAL EXPRESSIONS (examples)
First-person perspective Experienced continuity of life Experience of body	Basic assumptions World view Faith/Beliefs	Purpose in life Sense of significance Sense of coherence Belonging/Connectedness	Happiness/grief
Existential well-being **Suffering/joy of life**	Attitudes to the body Relation to nature	Engagement/Existential indifference Curiosity Hope Existential loneliness	Social attitudes Political viewpoints Religious attitudes Life philosophy
Sense of meaning *Crisis of meaning*	*Sources of meaning*	*Lived meaning* Quality of life	*Life decisions*
Identity feeling Self-image	Basic acceptance	Self-confidence Guilt and shame	Some personality traits
Dream life Art impressions Longing Visions	Flexibility/rigidity in orientations	Inner homeostasis Autonomy/freedom Internal locus of control	Art expressions

Subjectivity ←————————————————————→ Manifestation

- *Sources of meaning*, which are considered the subjectively recognisable areas where meaning is created or derived for the individual;
- *Lived meaning*, which is the quality of active involvement in life; meaningful living. Lived meaning can be further divided into four topics on which lived meaning is based: coherence, significance, orientation (purpose), and belonging.

Following the line of thought in this chapter and throughout the whole book, the logical next step can be a broad statement of what existential health is all about:

Existential health is the well-being and the well-functioning of the existential components.

If this statement is seen as a proposal for a definition of existential health, the proposal will be as broad and fluffy as the other definitions of physical, mental, and social health, and it will include the same key words of well-being and well-functioning as the other definitions.

The next chapters will look into empirical and practical approaches to the existential elements, hopefully making them more relevant for health seen as a whole. We can find empirical links between some of the existential components and other kinds of health, thereby bringing them into play with the complexity of our shared world, and can see what findings might be of interest in relation to other dimensions of health.

7

EMPIRICAL CONNECTIONS

Existential health and other health dimensions

Modern health science demands evidence for everything. When it comes to existential health, the same demand will be made. Is existential health really healthy? How do we measure whether it is healthy?

Part of this question is absurd and self-evident, but other parts of the question could be very constructive, allowing us to focus on some research that has been known for a long time, but somehow considered of minimal relevance to health. As will be shown, this is not the case.

First, the absurd and self-evident part of the question. Since health is largely defined as well-being, it is absurd to ask whether existential health is part of health. Existential health is the only dimension of health that includes well-being, because well-being is a subjective experience. One cannot talk about well-being without also talking about a person experiencing it. Well-being is the goal of all other health efforts, whether physical, mental, or social. No subject, no human health.

The same is not the case with the later definition of health as a resource for functioning well (see Chapter 1.2.3). In this line of definition, we can talk about health as processes that support experiences of well-being, the machinery of bodily processes, learning capabilities, and a benevolent social environment, not including any conscious knowledge about the functioning or feeling of well-being.

With the picture of the four-dimensional model, we can ask whether there is any evidence, that is, signs of interaction, that existential health contributes to good exchange and integration with the other dimensions of health. In other words: Does good existential health contribute to health changes in other dimensions, and can we build some ideas about a causal relationship between the dimensions, suggesting existential health to contribute with more than the experience of well-being?

Following the order of the existential map (previous chapter), this chapter will give a brief overview of known empirical findings. As health is a multifaceted

DOI: 10.4324/9781003502364-9

concept and as the health literature is vast, only a few important results will be mentioned, with a tendency to favour the simplest and most reliable measure of bad health: mortality. For the existential dimension, we will start in reverse order with the easiest to measure, the existential health expressions.

7.1 Existential expressions and health correlates

7.1.1 Is it healthy to be happy?

For many, happiness may be close to the very goal of life itself, and seen as such, the question is almost meaningless. But in other perspectives, it could be a good question. Do happy people live longer and with less disease?

Serious research has been looking at this for decades, and the answer is a big yes! – along with the opposite result of unhappiness contributing to bad health: 'Impaired happiness is not only a consequence of ill-health but also a potential contributor to disease risk' (Steptoe, 2019, p. 41).

Once this is said, the complexity of the question opens up: What kind of happiness? What kind of good health? A lot of complex and inconsistent findings have to be addressed, and the right research question might rather be if, why, and when subjective well-being (or happiness) influence health (Diener et al., 2017). Happiness is simply too diverse a concept to say anything simple about. The contemporary reviews all note the complexity of the research that has been done in the field.

A recent review article (Mendes et al., 2023) summarises that there is a 'significant body of research independently associating the presence of happiness and well-being with a lower risk of mortality and with improved physical and mental health status' (p. 288), but then immediately goes on with a long list of 17 overlapping concepts related to and overlapping the terms 'happiness' and 'well-being,' such as for example flourishing, positive affect, affect balance, life satisfaction, and quality of life. What is to be included, what is to be excluded?

A major distinction in the understandings of the term 'happiness' that is found almost everywhere in the recent literature is the distinction between hedonic well-being and eudaimonic well-being (Baumeister et al., 2013; Ryff & Singer, 2008). Hedonic well-being is understood as the maximisation of pleasure, the achievement of goals and cherished outcomes, and the minimisation of negative and unpleasant feelings. It is seen as the opposite of eudaimonic well-being, which is described as the fulfilment of one's true potential in terms of meaning and purpose in life. The effects of the two types of happiness are not alike.

When happiness is defined in smaller units, it seems easier to show clear results. A longitudinal study of American and Japanese samples found that happiness, understood as greater life satisfaction, higher positive affect, and lower negative affect, independently (i.e. controlled for other known contributors to health) improved health, reduced the prevalence of chronic health conditions, and lowered the risk of mortality (Willroth et al., 2020).

One problem with this kind of research is that it is not known which way the causality runs. Good health might lead to greater happiness, and great happiness might lead to good health. We need prospective studies to solve this problem, and there are quite a substantial number of them also (Chida et al., 2009). Recent critical articles do not question this fact, but they do raise the next question: How can we understand the pathways from happiness to physical health? Some very plausible such pathways are suggested as 1) neurobiological processes, 2) the indirect impact on health behaviour, 3) the promotion of protective psychosocial resources, and 4) stress-buffering effects (Mendes et al., 2023).

Does unhappiness lead to poorer physical health? As noted above, the answer is again a yes (e.g. Rovner, 1991). An animal study of this phenomenon examines mortality in animals in the light of past negative affect and suggests pathways via continuous activation of the hypothalamic-pituitary-adrenal and sympathetic-adreno-medullary axes, leading to increased mortality (Walker et al., 2012).

7.1.2   Religion, political orientation, and health

A large and growing body of research has been dedicated to the relationship between religion and health. There is strong evidence for an association, particularly studied in the US. An impressive review of over 1,200 research articles is provided by Harold Koenig and colleagues in the comprehensive *Handbook of Religion and Health* (second edition) (Koenig et al., 2012). Positive associations (good health) are found between religious involvement and the following mental health categories: well-being and positive emotions, depression, suicide, anxiety disorders, psychotic disorders, alcohol and drug abuse, delinquency and crime, and marital instability. In the case of physical health, better health for the religiously involved is found in these categories: heart disease, hypertension, cerebrovascular disease, Alzheimer's and dementia, immune function, endocrine function, cancer, mortality, physical disability, pain and somatic symptoms, health behaviour, and disease prevention.

Some of the research referred to in the book seems to have a somewhat typical American missionary tendency towards Christianity and can be – and has been – discussed in many ways, but growing research is secular based (European), and basic findings are also replicated in Muslim cultures.

Among the most robust findings are the association between church attendance and longevity – also in secular environments (Chida et al., 2009; la Cour et al., 2006) – and the relationship between religion and depression. Religious attendance seems to buffer the tendency to get depressed (Braam et al., 2001), and for the already depressed, and it seems to better the chances and time used for recovery (Koenig et al., 1998).

Organised religion and the consequences such as church attendance might be accused of actually measuring other things such as social engagement, physical activity, and the like that are known to be connected to physical health, so it is noteworthy that the studies control for as many of these covariates as possible. Even in very secular Denmark, a low rate of church attendance (more than two times a year) prolonged the lifespan by nearly two years for elderly at the age of 70 when primary data was recorded and followed over 20 years. The association was controlled for age, gender, functional ability, self-rated health, chronic conditions, depression, anxiety, marital status/living alone, social contact frequency, help given to others and received by others, smoking, alcohol, and Body Mass Index, and was still significant (la Cour et al., 2006).

It is still debated whether spirituality, agnosticism, and atheism are associated in the same way as religion. The results seem much more diverse in these areas, often indicating that questions of existential uncertainty (quest) might play a negative role concerning other health dimensions. It is consistently found that religious struggles are associated with poorer health (Fitchett et al., 2004; Pargament et al., 2001).

Much less research has been done on other ways of orientating one's life, such as political attitudes and life philosophies. Some relations have been suggested, but the field is not uniform, as health does not always follow the usual political divisions into left and right. Health is related to health behaviors, but health behaviors are often related to other political dividing lines than left and right.

In earlier times, a simple logic of conservatives being more economically wealthy and therefore having longer life expectancy could be affirmed, but during recent decades, it has been a pattern in the Western world, or at least in the US, that morbidity and mortality are due to health behaviours and lifestyle to a greater extent than environmental conditions (wealth), medical care, social circumstances, and genetics (Kannan et al., 2018). The direction of the association has now changed, and conservatism is now generally seen as connected to a less healthy lifestyle: conservatives eat fewer servings and varieties of fruits and vegetables, eat more high-fat and processed food, are less interested in health information, have lower odds of flu vaccination, and exercise less. On the liberal side, higher odds of cigarette smoking and excessive drinking were found (Kannan et al., 2018).

During the Covid-19 period, the relationship between political ideology and health behaviours was intensively studied. In the US, a study found political ideology to be the most significant predictor of most Covid-19-related health behaviours, including risk perception and vaccination intention, and concluded that political ideology is an important social determinant of health (Geana et al., 2021). In the same vein, a recent study found associations between political views and health literacy (an individual's ability to find, understand, and use health information) during the Covid-19 epidemic (Cameron et al., 2023). Health literacy during the Covid-19 period was associated with adaptive beliefs, attitudes, and behaviours;

greater concern for society; and less risky behaviour. The results showed that health literacy was positively associated with liberal political views, to a lesser extent with moderate views, and was weaker or absent with more conservative views.

Causality in the other direction – from health to political orientation – is also scarce and appears to be random across topics. Among the findings are that people with poor health are found to be more open to and more likely to use complementary/ alternative medicine (Valtonen et al., 2023), and a recent study found that children with excellent health in childhood are more likely to have a conservative than a liberal ideology as adults. The study does not control for whether children with excellent health are over-represented in wealthy families, which tend to be more conservative, and that the causal link, therefore, could be ordinary social learning from conservative parents.

7.1.3   Life decisions and health

Some important decisions in life have lasting consequences for how the rest of our lives will be shaped – including our health – although this is rarely the reason why these decisions are made. Such important decisions are usually perceived as free, independent choices made by the individual, although there might be questions of a philosophical, psychological, and sociological nature about whether such decisions are truly free and personal.

In any case, most people will experience things like their choice of education and profession as their own choice, their choice of marriage and to whom, their choice of whether or not to have children, their choice of where to live, and at the end, the personal choice about the possibility of taking one's own life, whether that choice is formulated as suicide, assisted suicide, euthanasia, or other variations on the theme.

Some review articles in the area of life choices and health are briefly mentioned below.

The choice of education and later working life has a very great influence on health; links between *education* and health have been an established fact for decades (von dem Knesebeck et al., 2006). Higher levels of educational attainment are consistently associated with better health outcomes and longer life expectancy, and to an astonishing degree. Each year of education is associated with a 2% lower mortality risk, and education of 18 years or more is associated with a 34% lower risk of dying early (Balaj et al., 2024). The pathways and many covariates in this association are widely discussed. Usually, economic factors, societal determinants, and inequality in education possibilities are mentioned as mediators for the association (Zajacova & Lawrence, 2018), giving opportunities for political initiatives.

Even with the same years of education, however, there are differences between *jobs* and careers. For example, the medical profession is known to have a fairly large impact on lifetime expectancy, with doctors dying up to 10 years earlier than other comparable groups and having higher suicide rates (Brayne et al., 2021; Pandey & Sharma, 2019).

There are also strong associations between *marriage* and health. Overall, being married is very healthy in terms of both physical and mental health (Robles, 2014; Robles et al., 2014). Married individuals have lower rates of morbidity and mortality from several health issues, including heart disease and cancer, and they report lower levels of depression. The positive effects of marriage are strongest for men.

Having *children* is also associated with better health (Modig et al., 2017) for both men and women. In Sweden, life expectancy at age 60 is two years longer for men and one and a half years longer for women, and the risk of cancer is also lower for women.

Choosing where to live has an impact on health as well. Life choices such as moving abroad for longer periods of life are likely to have consequences related to the different environments and health systems in different countries. Living in different places in the same country also affects health, although in different directions in different countries. In England, a study showed a greater life expectancy when living in rural districts than in urban areas (Kyte & Wells, 2010), while the opposite is true in the US, where rural residents live shorter lives (Walker & Brown, 2022).

As a living subject, every individual has to deal with the possibility of *suicide* – often perceived as the final solution to personal problems. Suicide has a place in the official mortality statistics and is, of course, an element of public health as well as mental and sociological health, but in the end, it is still the individual, the subject, who makes the decision on his or her own behalf. It is a fatal life decision. It reflects very poor existential health, where suffering overrides the will to live, and life is judged not worth living. In that sense, suicide hotlines and suicide teams in psychiatry are examples of urgent existential first aid units.

Suicide is not that rare; it happens about 100 times per million per year in Europe and nine per million in the US. In Europe, the suicide rate among men is, alarmingly, almost four times higher than among women.

Another kind of suicide that goes outside the official statistics is *assisted suicide*, which today is legal in some countries. The topic is under growing public debate in all Western countries and the debate is growing, and the number of completed assisted suicides has been ever-rising in the countries that allow it.

Assisted suicide might be the prime example of subjective considerations of a life worth living: when is death the better alternative? If we set aside the arguments in the debate about the possible misuse of euthanasia (relatives slightly pushing the decision etc.), the individual as a subject has to weigh the pros and cons of life itself in all its complexity – emotional, social, physical, economic, practical, and all other considerations that might be important in the single case. Existential decisions cannot be reduced to a simple formula, nor can existential help and support.

It is the political system that makes assisted suicide possible through legislation, but it is the health system that is responsible for the practical implementation of the decision. In addition to all the personal and social considerations, it involves trained health professionals at several levels, all of whom are involved by their own ethical considerations about actively participating in taking the life of another person. A reasonable question might be to ask how well prepared are health professionals as individuals to make the ethical and conscious decision about their personal cooperation in assisted suicide. Are they all on their own?

7.1.4   *Personality traits and health*

According to modern personality psychology, some personality traits are very hardwired into our brains and bodies. Research on the 'big five' (five personality traits that are said to be the same all over the world) has shown predictable relations with health. The personality trait Conscientiousness is associated with better health through engagement in health behaviours; Neuroticism is associated with worse health through emotional instability and anxiety; and Extroversion, Agreeableness, and Openness are associated with better health through better social engagement (Cao & Ji, 2024).

Other personality traits may not seem as hardwired, but rather dependent on life experiences and life considerations of a more subjective nature that are built into the personality through habits, life events, and social roles (Wagner et al., 2020). An example of such a trait might be generosity. This trait has been found to be very positively associated with both mental and physical health (Smith & Davidson, 2014). It is associated with lower levels of depression and anxiety, improved self-esteem, and better social connectedness, and for those who are engaged in voluntary work, it is found to be associated with longevity (Rogers et al., 2016).

7.2   Existential qualities and health correlates

Following the backwards order from right to left on the existential map (Table 6.1) the next step is the category of existential qualities. These qualities are less visible and less measurable than the existential expressions because they are closer to the subjective experience and less expressed. Nevertheless, some of the themes have been researched in relation to other dimensions of health.

7.2.1   *Meaning and health*

The topic of meaning in life is very broad and needs to be broken down into smaller pieces, depending on which aspects are meant in each case. There have been several attempts to measure aspects of meaning in life through questionnaires. Different questionnaires use a wide spectrum of understandings and wording. Historically, some of the main measurement scales can be named: Purpose in Life test (PIL)

(Crumbaugh & Maholick, 1964); Sense of Coherence Scale (Antonovsky, 1993a); Meaning in Life Questionnaire (Steger et al., 2006); Sources of Meaning in Life Questionnaire (SOME) (Schnell, 2009).

Although the measurements are different, the results all point in the same direction: Meaning in life is healthy. In a comprehensive review of meaning and health from 2014, Roepke et al. (2014) take the trouble to distinguish between six different understandings of the concept of meaning used in questionnaires. Combining all six, they use *meaning as an overall concept* and review a total of 62 articles on the topic. The overall results are very clear: Meaning in life is overall very beneficial for health. The benefits of meaning in life include

> faster recovery from surgery, lower risk of disability in old age, greater odds of survival from HIV, cancer, and myocardial infarction, greater longevity, better immune function, better regulation of the autonomic nervous system, and better subjective health and health-related quality of life. (p. 1068)

They also found that people with more meaning were more likely to engage in health-promoting behaviours such as exercise, non-smoking and so forth, which might explain some of the relationships between meaning and health. These positive effects were not found for people searching for meaning, which might be an older term for having a crisis of meaning.

Another, but smaller, systematic review of a broad mix of meaning scales and health was conducted in 2017 and found that the strongest relationships between meaning and health were found when meaning is measured with combined items of peace and well-being, compared to those that only focused on meaning in life (Czekierda et al., 2017). This finding opens up a critical perspective on these studies, that is, whether the meaning questionnaires also include items of well-being, as any item of well-being will naturally be highly correlated with well-being questionnaires. There is a risk that questions with the same content will be answered twice in two different questionnaires, leading to false conclusions of high associations between the results.

7.2.2   Purpose in life and health

When breaking meaning down into different types of meaning, we can better track what is actually being asked. The Purpose in Life test (PIL) has been very well studied, and because it is an old questionnaire dating back to 1964, some longitudinal studies have been possible, following the same people over decades.

One such longitudinal study was conducted in 2015 on all-cause mortality and cardiovascular events (heart attacks) (Cohen et al., 2015). More than 130,000 people were included in the study. A significant association was observed between having a higher purpose in life and reduced all-cause mortality (adjusted relative risk 0.83) as well as cardiovascular events. This is a very impressive result, but without the possibility to further investigate the moderators, the bridges of causality.

Causality was more visible in a 2018 cross-sectional study that analysed data from over 15,000 people (Musich et al., 2018). They found that purpose in life was strongly associated with social support, resilience, resilience in faith, high health literacy, and good health status. They also found significantly lower healthcare use and spending, higher adherence to preventative services compliance, and a higher quality of life among those who scored medium and high on the Purpose in Life test.

In the 2014 systematic review mentioned above (Roepke et al., 2014), purpose in life is reported to be associated with specifics such as better perceived health among cardiac patients and caregivers of people with cancer, but also with more general health tendencies towards better or even optimal sleep. In fibromyalgia patients, purpose in life was associated with higher pain tolerance and lower physical disability. Among very objectified health measures, purpose in life was associated with better recovery from knee surgery, fewer post-mortem neuronal changes in Alzheimer's disease, a lower risk of death from cardiovascular disease, and greater six-year survival among heart transplant patients.

7.2.3 Sense of coherence and health

Sense of coherence has been a term with a rather fixed content due to the extensive theoretical work of Aaron Antonovsky in the 1980s and the scale he developed (Antonovsky, 1993b; Antonovsky & Sagy, 1986). As a stress researcher, his main thought was that a sense of coherence is a buffer against stress. The term 'salutogenesis' (what develops health) was coined, and he had very strong hopes and theories about how the sense of coherence would be a major contributor to both physical and mental health. The theories were based on standard cognitive theories of stress and coping at the time (Eriksson, 2022). The theory of sense of coherence was very popular and recognised in hundreds of books and articles. However, the empirical data supporting and validating the theory did somehow not appear in the speed and quantity expected, and after 10 years the first critical signs showed up (Eriksson & Lindström, 2005). The much-hyped Sense of Coherence Scale was still labelled as 'stable' but not as stable as Antonovsky had originally assumed. It turned out not to be inconsistent in measuring what was intended to be measured, and the results were divergent. Reviews of findings at that time found that the scale was good at correlating to some psychological parts of stress, but failed to show any strong association with physical health aspects (Flensborg-Madsen et al., 2005). Another decade later, a large systematic review among adolescents again found sense of coherence associated with psychological elements such as quality of life, mental health, and family relationships, with no mention of physical health (Länsimies et al., 2017). Proponents of the popular theory were clearly disappointed by the continued lack of positive findings. The reason for that seems mainly to be found in the lack of quality of the scale used to measure it – the original Antonovsky scale. Recent validation of the scale in other languages has found that the psychometric properties of the scale are simply poor (Sebo et al., 2024).

Sense of coherence is a famous concept, which is why the rather poor research results in relation to health are mentioned here. Antonovsky's scale has so far monopolised research on the subject of sense of coherence, and we must hope that a better developed instrument will emerge.

7.2.4 Quality of life and health

A recent, very convincing systematic review and meta-analysis shows consistent results relating quality of life to health (Phyo et al., 2020). Using a variety of instruments measuring the quality of life and covering data from a total of 1.2 million participants, it concludes that a better quality of life is associated with a lower risk of death.

Looking more closely at what is called the health-related quality of life (measured by the scale SF36), it is found that it is the measures of physical functioning and general mental health that are most associated with lower mortality.

These findings may seem a little odd to include in a book that otherwise argues that quality of life, as an existential quality, should not be seen as a means to health but as an end in itself. But one small detail is worth noting: It is the *well-functioning* of the physical and mental aspects of quality of life that is most strongly associated with lower mortality risk. This lends some support to the previous statement that well-functioning and well-being are closely connected.

A critical comment might be that it is difficult to judge the causal pathways in this type of research: Is it the quality of life that leads to more years of life, or is it the well-functioning physical and mental capacities that lead to a better quality of life?

7.2.5 Locus of control and health

The term 'locus of control' is a rather old psychological concept, coined and instrumentalised by psychologist Julian Rotter in 1954. He theorised that people can have different beliefs in their own actions and decisions. Some believe that their own behaviour has a strong influence on what happens in their life, called the internal locus of control, while others believe that their lives are mostly influenced by factors such as fate, luck, and powerful others, called the external locus of control.

It might seem surprising that what on the surface appears to seem like rather small differences in attitudes have large associations with illness and death, but they have. A recent, large study followed more than 25,000 people for eight years starting in 2008 (Lindström et al., 2022). The external locus of control was significantly associated with more deaths from any cause, even after adjustment for socio-demographic factors and chronic disease. After adjustment for health-related behaviours (smoking, alcohol consumption, exercise, and intake of vegetables and fruits), the association between external locus of control and death was reduced but still present.

One might wonder why this difference in attitude seems so powerful. It may be because this attitude is closely related to other existential qualities such as self-confidence, autonomy, and a sense of significance. Research into these other components has not yet been conducted.

7.2.6   Loneliness and health

It is difficult to distinguish between different types of loneliness, but the authors of a 2012 study (Luo et al., 2012) tried their best by controlling their data on loneliness for the number of social relationships. They discovered that their main finding, that loneliness was associated with increased mortality, could not be explained by the number of social relationships, nor by health behaviours. Subsequent studies have found a gender difference, with lonely men having a higher mortality than lonely women (Henriksen et al., 2019). This finding has been replicated in a large meta-analysis (Rico-Uribe et al., 2018), which concludes that loneliness has a harmful effect on all-cause mortality and that the effect is slightly stronger for men than for women.

7.3   Life orientations and health correlates

Still moving from right to left on the map of existential components, we come next to the group under the heading life orientations. According to the framework, this group of components is less manifested, more subjective, and thereby less visible to others. Research will therefore need to focus on what can be seen as derivatives of the components, rather than the components in themselves.

7.3.1   Attitudes to the body and health

As seen above, a major factor in explaining physical and mental health is what is known as health behaviours. This is a broad term usually connected to highly visible and measurable things such as not smoking, the limiting of alcohol intake, time spent for exercise, and eating habits that lead to being overweight. In more recent research, food intake is more finely measured by the amount of greens and fruit.

All this can be said to refer to the subjective attitude to one's own body. Health behaviours are mostly subjective choices made in order to preserve and maintain a healthy body with less risk of disease and suffering. They are life choices made from the basic orientation system, the basic attitudes towards the body. In the case of dietary preferences, the life choice to be a vegetarian may also be dependent on the attitude towards nature, in this case, the animals that live with us, or on the ecology of the planet.

Health behaviours are extremely beneficial to health. That is why we call them health behaviours. Reference to any specific research might mainly knock down open doors. So just a few: A special issue of the journal *Psychology and Health* was dedicated to health behaviours and looked into the challenges of promoting future health behaviours, meaning illness prevention (Conner & Norman, 2017). Good health behaviours are not only for physical health. One study showed that changed health behaviour also improved subjective well-being over a long period (Stenlund et al., 2022). Vast health benefits from vegetarianism are known, including lower mortality (Key et al., 1999).

The Seventh-Day Adventists are a Christian group that maintains many health behaviours for religious reasons. They do not smoke; drink alcohol, black tea, or coffee; or eat meat; and they exercise. It has long been known that this group lives significantly longer than the general population. A study in California showed that men lived 7.3 years longer and women 4.4 years longer (Fraser & Shavlik, 2001). For strict vegetarians, the extended life expectancy was even longer.

7.3.2 Basic acceptance and health

The theme of acceptance of suffering as a basic remedy is being systematised and explored in the Acceptance and Commitment movement of psychotherapy (ACT) (Hayes et al., 2003). Initial acceptance of suffering from things that cannot be changed has been the aim of treatment for living with chronic illness conditions of various kinds: pain, disability, cancer, arthritis, and the like. Acceptance-focused attitudes in treatment are often compared with the older cognitive-based and control-focused attitudes (Szcześniak et al., 2020).

Research on acceptance attitudes has been aided by the presence of different acceptance of illness-scales, such as the Chronic Pain Acceptance Questionnaire (Vowles et al., 2009). Along with chronic illness conditions, acceptance (as addressed in ACT) has also been shown to be beneficial for mental disorders such as depression and for better cognitive function in general, and recently it has been found to increase psychological flexibility in general (Liu et al., 2023).

7.3.3 Sources of meaning and health

Research on different sources of meaning and health is still to come, but a study has been done on how working with and exploring personal sources of meaning affects chronic pain (Böhmer et al., 2022). The study is small and can only serve as an appetiser in this context. Forty-two patients with chronic pain were randomised, and the treatment group received a one-hour intervention aimed at getting the patients to explore their own sources of meaning in more detail, bringing the personal sources into focus in a structured conversation (the SoMCaM method, see la Cour & Schnell, 2020). Compared with the control group, which received standard care only, the intervention group showed a large increase in pain acceptance; a decrease in anxiety, depression, and crisis of meaning; and even a reduction in the pain intensity. The effect sizes were medium to large, meaning there was a substantial difference between the two groups.

7.3.4 Flexibility/rigidity and health

As mentioned above, ACT has been found to enhance psychological flexibility as a benefit of basic acceptance. In that way, also patterns of mental patterns of suffering can be altered, and the increased flexibility has been shown to have an effect on PTSD and trauma-related symptoms (Rowe-Johnson et al., 2024). The same mechanism of enhanced mental flexibility might also be the causal link for the research showing that work with acceptance has an effect on depression (Zhao et al., 2023). In recent psychology, psychological flexibility has been described as a fundamental aspect of health itself (Kashdan & Rottenberg, 2010).

In a recent study of the use of complementary/alternative medicine in 19 European countries, the research group extended the traditional left–right political dimension to include attitudes of green/alternative/libertarian orientations versus traditional/authoritarian/nationalist orientations. This dimension can also be perceived as a flexibility/rigidity dimension and is thus close to the existential component of basic life orientations. The researchers found that the green, alternative, and liberal political orientations were more likely to use complementary/alternative medicine (CAM) than the traditional, authoritarian, and nationalist orientations (Valtonen et al., 2023). The use of CAM can be viewed in different ways. Biomedical views are often negative, as they perceive the alternative as a threat to the established health organisations, questioning their authority. Another view could be that CAM use is an attempt to look at life in a more holistic way, which often corresponds to the choice of certain lifestyles, usually more health-oriented lifestyles with integrated health behaviours. This was the finding of a big American study with 35,000 participants (Bishop et al., 2019). The authors found that 45% of CAM users were motivated by CAM therapies to make positive health behaviour changes, and that many of the CAM therapies themselves involved such behaviour changes, especially changes in diet.

7.4 Subjective experience of living and health correlates

The last group of components (experience of living) might be difficult to relate to other kinds of health that can be measured, as this group is defined as the essence of subjectivity. However, known research can be seen as very close to two of the components.

7.4.1 Subjective self-rated measures and health

The basic experience of being in a body is one component. Subjectively, we scan the body all the time, and if something alarms the body feeling, it gets our attention. Basically, we just have a sense of being situated in the body, and the body can be perceived as having a basic neutral tone of well-being most of the time.

When asked: 'In general, would you say your health is…', and given the answer possibilities of 'excellent,' 'very good,' 'good,' 'fair,' and 'poor,' everyone seems to be able to answer, and this is how self-rated health is measured in the SF36 questionnaire. Surprisingly, this very simple question about how the subjects rate the health of their own body, shows impressively consistent results as an independent predictor of mortality (Idler & Benyamini, 1997). The prediction of mortality measured by self-rated health is even better than objective health risk predictions (Reinwarth et al., 2023). The subjective experience of the body must somehow contain some unexpressed sense of predictive value that goes beyond conscious knowledge. We are in an area where a sense of holism as the basic mode of recognition might be most pronounced.

7.4.2 Near-death experience and health

The other component where known research can be applied is the near-death experience. As most people know, this is a possible universal experience for the human race in situations where personal death is very close. It is not rare. About 10%–18% of people who survive cardiac arrest can report such an experience. It has been reported since ancient times and from all over the world (Greyson, 2022). The experience can vary on certain themes, but usually, there is an out-of-body experience where the present (death) situation is viewed from elsewhere, typically from above. Sometimes, there is an experience of the personal life being reviewed in a different time perspective, and sometimes, there are reports of encounters with close, deceased family members and with mystical beings.

The near-death experience is reported to have a major impact on the view of life in the years following and on the fear of death. When interviewed a few months after the experience, survivors often express a completely new meaning of life and death (Zingmark & Granberg-Axèll, 2022), and measured with a scale called the Life Changes Inventory, these changes in attitudes towards life and death are persistent over at least two decades (Greyson, 2022). Especially for the fear of death, experiences of encounters with mystical beings appear to be the strongest predictor of changed attitude, while the sense of disembodiment is not associated with change in attitudes (Pehlivanova et al., 2023).

As noted in the literature, these experiences may bear some resemblance to psychedelic experiences, which have seen a great resurgence of research in recent years (Barber & Aaronson, 2022). Psychedelic therapy has shown surprisingly good effects on post-traumatic stress disorder (PTSD), depression, alcohol and drug abuse, anxiety, and end-of-life care (Mitchell & Anderson, 2023). This research emphasises that it is not the actual chemical drug used that causes the effect and change (as in conventional pharmaceutical medicine), but the subjective experiences themselves. Again, there is explanatory attention to the effects directed towards heightened flexibility in attitudes, sometimes referred to as neuroplasticity (Kishon et al., 2024).

It can be argued that such research findings might not be of essential value in a biomedical view of health, but rather of value for the existential health itself. Such considerations may be good examples of the limitations of the dominant biomedical or physical perspective on health, which in our modern society turns people into things and corpses rather than seeing them as human beings with a unique human potential to explore and enjoy life.

8

WHERE THE PRESENCE OF EXISTENTIAL HEALTH IS ALREADY EVIDENT

Throughout this book, various examples have been given of where the concept of existential health is at stake, and where its recognition and an emerging scientificity seem obviously justified. The somewhat scattered examples will be systematised here without, however, providing any comprehensive overview of where existential health is important. The general idea is that existential health will always be present in any encounter with the health system. Existential health will always be a dimension that can or should be included. Therefore, the following examples are more in the nature of places where existential health has obvious relevance.

8.1 Examples of relevant existential health concerns during the lifespan

Before individual life begins, it is a condition of modern society that the life of a newborn child is chosen, at least in the vast majority of cases. Someone, the biological mother and, in most cases, the father, has to make a life decision to have a child, that is, to stop using contraception and to engage in sexual intercourse or in artificial insemination processes. The *artificial insemination* processes are becoming more and more common, as the problem of infertility now affects one in six people worldwide according to the WHO (2023). It is a growing issue for healthcare systems, and failure to achieve success is deeply affecting the lives of the persons involved. The failure of the medical process cannot just be seen as a physical health problem of a technical nature, but as a new condition for living and the reorientation of meaning systems for the people hoping and striving to be parents. What might be a good educational background to be a partner in discussing the existential considerations of childless people?

DOI: 10.4324/9781003502364-10

The opposite, unwanted pregnancy, is also a practical task for healthcare. Legislation and availability of *abortion* are discussed in some places, abortion time limits in others, discussions which are always a matter of deep personal relevance to the pregnant girl or woman. Biomedical issues are only a small part of the decision to have an abortion. Counselling services exist in some form in most countries, but are not really part of medical organisation and medical education.

Childbirth itself is paradoxically found to increase awareness of death in new mothers, who are found to reflect on issues of their own finitude and the fragility of loved ones (Sejrsgaard et al., 2024). These openings to a deeper insight of life may be occurring naturally, but may not be met in a way that leads to personal growth and life acceptance of the mother. More research and creativity could be highly desirable.

Some children are born with physical or mental challenges, or develop them during childhood, some of which turn out to be serious *disabilities*. The children themselves are faced with different living conditions from others, and some might even doubt their status as full human beings. The carers of sick or disabled children may also find themselves in an unwanted position due to circumstances beyond their control, which have a major impact on their lives. Often their life orientations must change, and the need for ventilating and exchanging views on life can be seen in numerous websites and self-help books on the subject, but this need is not yet really seen as part of the official healthcare system. There is a documented need for help to maintain good resources and mental surplus for carers, leading to better life possibilities for both children and carers, and less use of costly institutional health services.

The Western world is currently experiencing a major *mental health crisis* of unhappiness, depression, and anxiety among young people, manifesting itself in various forms of borderline behaviour, including truancy, self-harm, use of painkillers, and occasionally suicidal thoughts (Keyes & Platt, 2024). This mental health crisis is not particularly psychiatric, and no one really knows what causes it; it seems to have emerged simultaneously at the same time as the Covid-19 isolation period. Causal links are suggested to be mainly of a social nature: social media and screen time, social isolation, climate change anxiety, social pressure to be perfect, and lack of mental health resources. All of these suggestions might have a common root related to problems of finding identity in contemporary society, a truly existential issue, but not addressed as such. It is troublesome to address it as an existential health issue because there is no common language for it and there is a lack of research on existential health issues.

At any point in life, the individual may face a life-threatening situation, such as undergoing major surgery, where future life conditions are in the hands of others and out of the individual's control. Serious *pre-surgery anxiety* has a prevalence of one in two. This needs to be addressed because pre-operation anxiety is linked with slower, more complicated and painful post-operative recovery, higher doses of pain medication, and, in the longer run, increased morbidity and mortality

(Bedaso et al., 2022). Some simple remedies are well known: Giving patients the opportunity to ask questions and talk during the preoperative period reduces the anxiety for 49% of patients, according to the same reference. The anxiety is not psychiatric, but a fully understandable, normal human existential response to a life-threatening condition. The lack of understanding and integration of such issues in almost any known surgical unit is also well known, and this example shows how much of a difference just a little integration of different health understandings could make. The point here is about making a humanistic conversation a prescribed possibility in the surgery unit.

As medical technology continues to expand, modern health considerations are also about the possibility of choosing between different health inventions. *Health choices* may be on the lighter end of the spectrum, such as the choice between dental intervention and replacement materials, which might be aesthetically relevant to one's self-image, or they might be heavily influenced by economic factors, for example in the choosing of quality of eyeglass lenses. However, health choices can also be on the very serious end, for example, where the professionals are unable to find any conclusive evidence about which intervention will serve the purpose best. It could be the choice of interventions in serious stages of cancer: One choice will *probably* give a better chance of survival with a low quality of life versus a choice of a probably lesser chance of survival with a lower level of side effects. The area of decision-making between options is well known and described as burdenful (Stacey et al., 2010).

This situation of patients making their own medical decisions has previously been discussed as a problem in the history of medicine. The crux of the problem has been when the patients disagreed with the remedy or medication decided by the physician, who in earlier times perceived themselves as unquestionable authorities. The most silent way to disagree with authority was simply not to take the recommended remedy as prescribed, which in older textbooks is called lack of *compliance*, while in newer textbooks, it is called lack of adherence. The patient, including the subjective sense of body and the personal orientation system, makes a choice of free will that is not taken into account by the medical profession. This, in a nutshell, is the problem of the lack of elaboration of the 'person' in the bio-psycho-social model.

The shift in language from compliance to adherence may be similar to the more modern view of medical authority. A further step down from the ivory tower may be the further development of *shared medical decision-making*, a term still mostly found in the literature related to the late stages of cancer. The healthcare system seems to have begun this fundamental recognition of the personal world of the patient by acknowledging that the decisions about personal health at the end of the day always will be the patient's own. That side of medical knowledge should be a future topic of research, and the building up of relevant skills for helping in making decisions on health should be mandatory in clinical health education, as it is a manifest area of existential health and healthcare.

That said, there are several dilemmas in taking the view of the patient seriously. The main one might be to balance patient autonomy with supposedly more rational healthcare decisions (Ilori et al., 2024). Individual preferences can be in opposition to what is known as best-evidence practice; the patient's decision might overtop what is practically and economically possible; the patient can have a limited capacity to make the decision on a well-informed basis. The views of the family may override what the patient thinks and believes. This is why there is a need for an expanded language, awareness, and education in the field.

The historical success of treatments and the expansion of the healthcare system mean that we are also becoming a society in which more and more people are living with one or more *chronic conditions*. A recent Canadian study found that 70% of the population live with one or more chronic conditions, and 45% live with multimorbidity (Steffler et al., 2021). In other words, most of us live with some form of disability, a chronic condition. Some of these conditions are well managed, such as by asthma medication, but others are very serious and involve suffering on a daily basis, such as chronic pain conditions, which are surprisingly common. In the Western world, around 20% of people are living with chronic pain, and 7% are significantly limited by pain in their daily activities (Nahin et al., 2023). Chronic pain is associated with severe depression, clinical insomnia, and a very low quality of life, like most of the chronic illnesses are. Chronic diseases are those that affect most people, and for the longest time.

It is a paradox that where there is the most disease, pain, and suffering present in a population, there is the least healthcare. When the diagnosis is made and there is no cure in sight, a few drugs may be introduced and prescribed to alleviate the symptoms, and then chronically ill patients are on their own, trying to manage a restricted life, often with a low quality of life and with a high degree of suffering. This is also the case for many cancer patients: Once the intensive cancer treatment is over, people are left on their own with very altered living conditions, having to struggle with a life worth living. For some illnesses, such as cancer and arthritis, there is often an outpatient clinic that offers a physical check from time to time and provides assistance if something changes physically, yet for other illnesses, there is no such outpatient service.

The art of finding and living a life of worth with a chronic disease could really benefit from more attention and research. It is well known that people with chronic conditions often struggle a lot to make their lives worth living, especially those patients suffering from diseases that attract very little medical interest, such as medically unexplained conditions. A study dares put a name to this special kind of suffering: the longing for existential recognition (Lind et al., 2014).

We can call the daily struggle for meaning in life many things: lack of quality of life, lack of meaning, purpose, significance, belonging, and hope. We can also call it very poor existential health, which may be a reasonable umbrella term. It is a huge health problem because it involves suffering for so many people, but it seems nearly invisible to the health system as it is organised today.

A good example of holistic health, including the existential perspectives, could be the *principles of person-centred care*. The idea of person-centred care is to see patients as individuals and equal partners in health services and to engage with patients with the principles of respect, dignity, and compassion held high. Other keywords are empowerment, continuity, and collaboration with families (Coulter & Oldham, 2016). So what is not to like? Nothing, but the fact that it is still mainly about principles and ideals and not about reality. The origins of the concept go back to humanism, but the naming of these ideas as person-centred can be traced back to around 2000, and from early on, we can find critiques of the term as being used rhetorically and with little practice behind it (Brooker, 2004). More recent articles look at the research and find almost none, but the few studies that have been done with person-centred care are positive. Clearly, better guidelines are needed on what defines person-centred care and to distinguish it from something that is not, in order to conduct relevant research (Marulappa et al., 2022).

Finally, in some areas of healthcare, the individuality of the client's world, the subject, the existential dimension, is at the centre of care because it is a necessity. These areas are related to the ending of life. In dementia, especially *severe dementia*, rational principles and logic must give way to following what is happening here and now for the patient. It is not possible to help patients to eat when they are furious. Many things must be timed and executed in a very flexible way to succeed. Trying to provide moments of joy for people living with severe dementia can be considered a creative dance by caregivers and staff to establish the right situation and moment for meaningful exchange and togetherness.

The next example of a place that takes an existential and holistic starting point is *suicide prevention services*, which may or may not be part of the official health system. Most often, such services are part of voluntary organisations. The public psychiatric units take care of the acute phases of unsuccessful suicides, often with a very technical attitude, such as assessing the current suicide risk when the patient is discharged from the unit. Somehow, it seems very strange that the official health system does not offer the best possible help in the prevention of suicidal plans and behaviour since death is seen as the primary enemy. On the other hand, this may also be the reason why suicide defies the logic that death is the biomedical worst case, and that is why biomedical-oriented systems are less equipped to manage and help such 'rebels.'

The final area to be mentioned here is that of *end-of-life care*, which could be nursing homes or hospices. Here, the focus is on the needs and preferences of the individual and their relatives, especially on the physical, mental, and social levels. Dying people are recognised and listened to if they want to smoke cigarettes, if they have special preferences for food and drink, and their social needs for companionship are met as far as possible. This is person-centred care in practice, based on compassion, respect, and collaboration. However, this is the case with one very strange exception: The existential dimension itself is rarely articulated. It could be supposed that end-of-life situations would be the natural place of existential thoughts about the life lived, the evaluation of it, the life choices made, maybe some regrets, and the recollection of the most wonderful periods of life – all this together with reflection on thoughts of death, philosophy of life, religiousness and other basic orientations. But according to research, staff rarely talk about these issues, although there is evidence that patients want to discuss existential issues with doctors and staff. A study done in the UK started from this fact (Abbas & Dein, 2011). The researchers asked staff members about barriers to discussing existential issues and listed the barriers as: lack of vocabulary around the issues, personal issues about death and dying, training issues, fear of being unable to resolve existential problems, time constraints, and difficulty in separating existential and religious needs.

This list of barriers could be a list of issues that need to be addressed in the training of any group of health workers if a culture change is to be achieved. Existential issues are as natural and common to humans as eating and kissing, but somehow we have developed a culture that is very afraid to talk about them openly.

8.2 Prevention of illness and existential health

Until about 1970, the biomedical perspective and methods alone defined what medical *science* was. In the following decade, several other perspectives from both sociology and psychology found common ground in a discipline called behavioural medicine (Pomerleau & Brady, 1979). The novelty of this approach is that it moves away from the medical clinical treatment situation as the basic method of medical knowledge and takes a broader view of illnesses as biologically, psychologically, and socially situated. Behavioural medicine fully embraces methods of sociology and psychology and brings topics such as health behaviour and health literacy into health science. The emerging new agendas are health promotion, prevention, and public health, aiming at specific diseases.

The type of psychology involved in this movement was called health psychology, which rejected the treatment situation as the source of knowledge about mental health. It valued empirical knowledge, which meant looking at people in groups, such as patient groups, work groups, or families (Ogden, 2012). It turned away from the non-empirical psychosomatic tradition and instead focused on how illness affected psychological well-being, mainly through empirical studies.

With a greater focus on large public health-orientated studies, behavioural medicine made a breakthrough in the causal explanations of diseases. Instead of monocausal and mechanical understandings of cause and effect, we all began to talk about risk factors, the increased likelihood of disease in groups of people. Preventative medicine moved from large community-based approaches such as sewage systems to the prevention of specific diseases in individual patients (Martin & Howell, 1989).

This is the kind of preventative medicine we know best today: knowledge from large amounts of data leading to advice on health behaviours. Preventative medicine was very active during the Covid-19 period when preventative medicine was also mixed up with health politics in a way that took it from health advice to legislation. More generally, however, the boundaries between what is health science and what is health politics are blurred. Many prevention initiatives have a large economic impact, particularly in reducing health costs for the population who are ill if they follow the health advice.

Anti-smoking campaigns are good examples of successful public health improvement and prevention initiatives. They reduce lung cancer and other specific diseases in individuals and have a large economic impact. Public health authorities also frequently give advice on nutrition (less fat etc.) and alcohol consumption. Some of this works well. It is a great public health success that life expectancy has increased as it has. In big statistics, it works; modern health service is a fantastic success. Good human health is, as said at the beginning of this book, a blessing for humanity, one of the most beautiful flowers of civilisation as we know it.

That said, there are still things to improve. There is more health to be gained through prevention, and the problem with big statistics is that they are about *the mean*. The mean is usually a number that expresses a kind of middle of a normal curve, where there is a part above the middle and a part below the middle. If we zoom in somewhere, there are movements that are not seen in the big picture. After an intervention, for example, there are usually some participants on the end below who have been worse during the intervention; their worsening is invisible if the mean has moved to the better. It is these participants who are relevant to focus on in a clinical setting, where persons are met person to person.

The same goes for prevention. We have statistics showing that smoking is decreasing in the general population, but some subgroups are increasing, and some individuals are in more danger of dying from smoking than others. Some are immune or resistant towards the general advice not to smoke. The advice and motivation are coming from the outside, the external.

The psychology of health behaviour change is traditionally of the cognitive/behavioural psychological orientation, focusing on observable thoughts and actions. It holds an external perspective on the human psyche, much like in pedagogy, and is based on principles of learning. A prominent example of such a model for behaviour change is called the Stages of Change Model (Prochaska & Velicer, 1997), which identifies five stages of change: 1) Pre-consumption, where there is no intention to act; 2) Contemplation, where there are intentions and plans to take action; 3) Preparation, where some steps towards action have been taken; 4) Action, where behaviour is changed for a short period of time; 5) Maintenance, where the behaviour has been changed and maintained for a longer period. Later models add the possibility of relapse and start from stage 2 again.

As seen, the model looks at and describes the individual from the outside, from the observer position. But when tobacco is available in society, quitting smoking is a truly personal question and decision. There has to be a subject who decides to stop smoking, who has to take up the fight with bodily cravings, and who has to put a higher principle of better health above the principle of hedonism and immediate needs fulfilment. It is an inner decision that leads to the actual smoke stoppage.

Seen this way, there may be limits to trying to get other people to change their health patterns from the outside without integrating the concrete subject who makes the decision. Ongoing alcohol and drug abuse and overweight reduction might be good examples of such limits; they are rarely changed by outside advice alone.

With the addition of the inner perspective, that is, the existential components, some other elements come into play. The importance of personal choice can be emphasised; it is a life decision. Life philosophies can be discussed in the context, the experience of the body, and the personal orientation system, including basic assumptions about the world and one's place in it. In this way, the choice of a health behaviour pattern can be seen as a personal choice in the direction of a life valued living. If the choice is made not to follow the advice, the choice can be open to others and perhaps also accepted as such without any judgemental attitudes.

In the end, any change in health behaviour will almost always be a subjective choice, and the choice of a healthy lifestyle is a life decision that can only be made by the individual. If talked about openly, it could also be respected as such, as we have different sources of meaning and different attitudes towards what constitutes a good life. For some, life is about enjoyment and fulfilment of needs – often referred to as a hedonistic life attitude – while for others, a good life is pursuit of personal growth, authenticity, and meaning – often referred to as a eudaemonic life attitude (Ryff & Singer, 2008).

9

SOME IMPLICATIONS OF EXISTENTIAL HEALTH

Throughout this book, health has been seen as essential to the good life. The good life is a life with sufficient health to live it. For this to be true, all dimensions of health need to be considered and integrated. However, such integration is not the case in modern healthcare, health research, and clinical health management.

The purpose of this book has not been to promote any particular discipline or mode of practice. Nor has it been the intention to promote any particular existential philosophy or psychology, although the thinking and some of the examples mentioned are from that school of thought.

The aim has been to enrich the field of health by trying to create better conditions for the necessary cultural change in healthcare and in understanding health. The culture change needs to move away from the atomised and technology-fixated understandings and instead look at what the goal of health really is. Health needs to be promoted as a whole, with the person whose health is at stake at the centre.

Change in society needs politics, plans, and ideas; it needs someone engaged to effect change, but it also requires a variety of resources to make the change possible. While a lack of resources in earlier times and in poor societies have related to the lack of material resources and remedies, the modern health system seems to have overgrown itself with technicalities, specialised knowledge, and tunnelling vision. The lack of resources in modern times seems to be of a different kind: the lack of overview and holism, a common idea and reflection. It is a lack of awareness of context.

The politics of contextual awareness is not something that can be brought in via a political programme, and it is not brought in from one year to another. In the context of existential health, the politics of this book have been some primary steps to enrich language and understanding with words, concepts, and models, with the purpose of continued thinking in this area. Without habit, the richness of language

DOI: 10.4324/9781003502364-11

and imagery in our minds, thoughts of existential health will become rare in our minds, and it will be harder to think along the lines of holism.

The easy thing is to do as usual, to do what is told by authority or soon what the AI data programme tells us to do. The choice is between what is good and what is easy, as it is said.

So, better words, better concepts, more thought, and more reflection on context in every health encounter are the health politics of this book. The remedies may be primarily related to health education programmes. A much more conscious attitude towards holistic health needs to be developed, which means respect for and knowledge of all types of education, specialities, branches, alternatives, and disciplines related to health. A culture needs to be developed in which it is possible to have specialists of several health dimensions to move in and out of each other's workspace, and in which incompetence in one health dimension does not mean that the patient is simply written off or discharged. Integrated health thinking must be a necessary first step to achieve this.

Fortunately, changes in this direction are already taking place. In part, this is because the integrated view on health was a virtue of some earlier medicine thinking. William Osler (1849–1919) talked about the good doctor being one skilled in both medicine and humanism, and this view might still have some active proponents who behave in accordance with both kinds of knowledge and are not blind to the broader context of the ill person. Some general physicians are actually still fighting for *the contextual attitude* (Shah & Foell, 2023).

Other shoots of contextualised health practice have grown from the bottom up out of necessity. There is the practice of person-centred care, for example, where it is fully practised. In palliative care and in the care of people with severe dementia, the context of reality is undeniably intrusive. Health advice, house rules, and regulations must give way to a more contextual view when the person wants to smoke a cigarette. In that context, even cigarettes are not unhealthy.

Such irregularities in formal health administration and glimpses of spontaneous integrated health thinking can also be found in mental health care, and thus maybe not fully consciously. In the care of people with Down syndrome, the existential dimension seems to be very prominent. Healthcare is about making life joyful and desirable for people with Down syndrome, who are usually cognitively and behaviourally impaired. Their impairment does not seem to matter so much as long as they possess enough cognitive abilities and functioning to serve a life valued of living.

Prevention, giving up old and building up new health behaviours can serve as a final example of possible contextual integration. For at least a hundred years, the treatment of drug and alcohol addiction has successfully integrated some existential components as active concepts. Keywords in addiction treatment books might be: acceptance of the condition of addiction, self-image, relation to nature and body, basic assumptions of life, purpose and meaning in life, internal locus of control, and finally, life decisions.

9.1 Training

The wish for a change in health learning and attitudes is, of course, helped by materials and language, but also by the skills, attitudes, and actions of those experienced in specific health disciplines. If it is natural to be aware and talk about the bigger picture in a workplace, then this overview will be more easily passed on to the younger people learning the discipline. Where this attitude and overview are absent, it will be very difficult for young students to get to know it and incorporate it when building their own professionalism. Inspiration, knowledge, and skills have to start somewhere. We simply need to incorporate talk on our common existential dimension on a daily basis, to learn the language to speak about it in a natural and relaxed way. It is not strange or unpleasant when learned. The content of existential education programmes and techniques for training existential conversation are most likely a topic for another whole book, but some sources for training can be mentioned briefly.

In the book *The Psychology of Meaning in Life* (Schnell, 2021), psychologist Tatjana Schnell devotes a significant part of the book to describing what she calls 'meaning-centred interventions.' She discusses different types of existential procedures and methods that can be learned by all health professionals. These include assistance in conducting life reviews in palliative care in both extended and short-term versions, and there are more aspirational sub-specialities, such as dignity therapy and cognitive reminiscence therapy. For those already familiar with the field, there is always the possibility of training and education in meaning-orientated or existential psychotherapies (Cooper, 2003; Van Deurzen & Arnold-Baker, 2005). Existential psychotherapy has been a long but rather narrow branch of psychotherapy for over a hundred years and has seen several varieties, including logotherapy and various subspecies, as for example meaningful living with cancer. The practice of existential psychotherapy may be close to what is practised in pastoral care (at least in the modern, open versions), both of which are seen as specialist professional tasks.

A new and much less demanding method of opening up the existential field of meaning in life to another person is the Sources of Meaning Card Method (la Cour & Schnell, 2020). The method is based on Schnell's extensive empirical work on sources of meaning and consists of a set of 26 cards with statements of possible sources of meaning in life. The standard exercise takes one hour to complete. The first stage of the method is for the person in focus to read and select the statements with which they feel most in tune as an individual. The next step is a semi-structured interview for each selected card in a two-person conversation. The procedure is easy to learn and can be used as training for future health professionals to talk in a normal conversational style about topics centred on meaning in life. The procedure increases and trains the ease with which health professionals can use words and terms of an existential nature (www.somecam.org).

As far as I know, there are no organised courses for health workers who want to improve their skills in existential interviewing and conversation, and that might be a sign of both the silence of the field and the shyness associated with it.

Basic conversational styles such as 'Socratic dialogue' are not well known or trained in mainstream health education, but would be of great help, especially the part about listening. Socratic dialogue is based on common human abilities and can be learned by everyone:

1. Asking open-ended questions that stimulate critical thinking
2. Practising active listening, where questions are built on the other person's responses
3. Critical questioning that challenges assumptions
4. Collaborative knowledge construction, where new insights and perspectives emerge through the dialogue

Why are these skills not trained for use in most health encounters and for all health workers?

9.2 'Physician, heal thyself'

The last part of Schnell's book on meaning in life is about meaning in work. She notes that the idea of finding personal meaning in one's work might be of recent origin, but it may be of particular interest here, as the working lives of health professionals are often the result of a personal choice to train in a helping profession and have a strong influence on the rest of their lives (Wedding & Stuber, 2020). In short, the healing professions often attract young people who wish to be of help in a close and concrete way, where inter-human relations are felt as important. For some, the years in medical school can be a process of desensitisation and disappointing training in technical attitudes. By the time these individuals enter the workforce, the question of meaning in work might arise with power, as the intentions of choosing a healthcare provider career and the actual work routines can seem far apart, and they may regret their carrier choice (Dyrbye et al., 2020; Khanfar et al., 2023).

Schnell (2021) identifies four themes as important to finding meaning in work:

1. The importance of the task. People need to feel that their daily tasks are important, that they make a difference that they can be proud of. When quantity comes before quality, the intrinsic meaning of work is easily forgotten.
2. A socio-moral atmosphere of belonging. The authoritarian leadership model does not create much meaning for employees, whereas an open, participative atmosphere creates employees with greater empathy, reliability, helpfulness, and solidarity according to empirical studies.

3. Self-transcendent organisations. Organisational goals such as maximising profit and efficiency are not really favoured by employees. Instead, values like solidarity and social responsibility are endorsed. The idea of the organisation having a 'higher purpose' has an inspiring, energising, and meaning-giving effect on the employees.
4. Work-role fit. The job needs to fit the person in terms of education, skills, personality, and interest in order to provide job satisfaction.

In this way, these points illustrate many of the shortcomings of modern healthcare, where management demands, for example in hospitals, focus on quantity, on authoritarian set targets for departments, on efficiency in achieving the targets set for the organisation, and on replacing staff where it suits the organisation. All are very illustrative of the situation of modern health workers, which seems to have further worsened in the aftermath of the Covid-19 pandemic (Barili et al., 2022; Galanis et al., 2023).

According to empirical studies, living a meaningful life is highly correlated with what Schnell calls vertical and horizontal self-transcendence (Schnell, 2011). In more general terms, this means the ability to reach out beyond oneself and engage in commitments and concerns beyond immediate self-interest. Meaning in life often follows such activities. Within this system of thought, meaning is related to a combination of purpose in life, significance, coherence, and belonging (Schnell, 2021). This is also true for health workers. If health work is reduced to mechanistic, efficiency-seeking, authoritarian actions, meaning is likely to be lost, and the existential health of the health workers themselves is at risk.

10

EPILOGUE

Health is a means, not an end. As suggested, the existential dimension can include, for example, thoughts of personal death, including the possibility of feeling 'full of days.' In this way, personal death can be 'death on time' and be embraced, and that would be a sign of existential health in action. Death is not the enemy, but the natural and healthy end. Death is essential for life on earth to continue; death has always been a necessity in evolution, an obligation of every creature; life would not have evolved if not for all the death creating new possibilities.

So, in this short period between our birth and our death, we may reflect on what brought us here without our knowing and what kind of end is possible. Existential concerns can lead us to strive for a good life, which is not a life of perfect health, but a life of sufficient health to make life worth living. The thoughts of evolutionary health might appear once more, the idea of layers of health emerging from each other, health seen as resources. As shown in Figure 10.1, the base will be the environmental and social health, which gives us the resources to have a body. Bodily health gives us the resources to have a mental life, and mental health gives us the resources to have an existential life. But if we follow this line of thought to the end: What is the existential life a resource for?

Here, my profession as a health psychologist has reached every limit and happily hands over the topic to philosophers and theologians, dreamers, politicians, activists, artists, and all living people with the resources and abilities to discover what life can be all about.

DOI: 10.4324/9781003502364-12

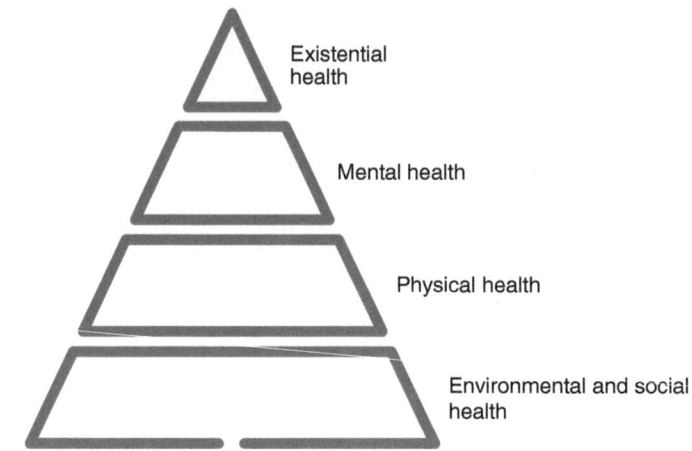

FIGURE 10.1   The pyramid of health seen as a resource.

REFERENCES

Abbas, S. Q., & Dein, S. (2011). The difficulties assessing spiritual distress in palliative care patients: A qualitative study. *Mental Health, Religion & Culture, 14*(3–4), 341–352.

Ahn, A. C., Tewari, M., Poon, C.-S., & Phillips, R. S. (2006). The limits of reductionism in medicine. *PLoS Medicine, 3*(6), e208. 10.1371/journal.pmed.0030209

Als, H. (1982). Toward a synactive theory of development: Promise for the assessment and support of infant individuality. *Infant Mental Health Journal, 3*(4), 229–243. 10.1097/PHM.0b013e31823d54be

Álvarez, A. S., Pagani, M., & Meucci, P. (2012). The clinical application of the biopsychosocial model in mental health: A research critique. *American Journal of Physical Medicine and Rehabilitation, 91*(13 Suppl. 1), 173–180. https://doi.org/10.1097/PHM.0b013e318 23d54be

Antonovsky, A. (1993a). The structure and properties of the sense of coherence scale. *Social Science and Medicine, 36*(6), 725–733. https://doi.org/10.1016/0277-9536(93)90033-Z

Antonovsky, A. (1993b). The structure and properties of the sense of coherence scale. *Social Science and Medicine, 36*(6), 725–733. https://doi.org/10.1016/0277-9536(93)90033-Z

Antonovsky, H., & Sagy, S. (1986). The development of a sense of coherence and its impact on responses to stress situations. *The Journal of Social Psychology, 126*(2), 213–225. https://search.proquest.com/openview/23b3e251ff80165fb8768c2bbaca33ce/1?pq-origs ite=gscholar&cbl=1819178

Balaj, M., Henson, C. A., Aronsson, A., Aravkin, A., Beck, K., Degail, C., Donadello, L., Eikemo, K., Friedman, J., Giouleka, A., Gradeci, I., Hay, S. I., Jensen, M. R., Mclaughlin, S. A., Mullany, E. C., O'connell, E. M., Sripada, K., Stonkute, D., Sorensen, R. J. D., … Gakidou, E. (2024). Effects of education on adult mortality: A global systematic review and meta-analysis. *The Lancet Public Health, 9*(3), e155–e165. https://doi.org/10.1016/S2468-2667(23)00306-7

Balzeau, A., Turq, A., Talamo, S., Daujeard, C., Guérin, G., Welker, F., Crevecoeur, I., Fewlass, H., Hublin, J. J., Lahaye, C., Maureille, B., Meyer, M., Schwab, C., & Gómez-Olivencia, A. (2020). Pluridisciplinary evidence for burial for the La Ferrassie 8 Neandertal child. *Scientific Reports, 10*(1), 1–10. https://doi.org/10.1038/s41598-020-77611-z

Barber, G. S., & Aaronson, S. T. (2022). The emerging field of psychedelic psychotherapy. *Current Psychiatry Reports, 24*(10), 583–590. https://doi.org/10.1007/S11920-022-01363-Y

Barili, E., Bertoli, P., Grembi, V., & Rattini, V. (2022). Job satisfaction among healthcare workers in the aftermath of the COVID-19 pandemic. *PLoS ONE, 17*(10 October). https://doi.org/10.1371/journal.pone.0275334

Bateson, G. (2013). Steps to an ecology of mind. In *Steps to an ecology of mind.* University of Chicago Press. https://doi.org/10.7208/chicago/9780226924601.001.0001

Batson, C. D., Schonrade, P., & Ventis, W. L. (1993). *Religion and the individual. A social-psychological perspective.* Oxford University Press.

Baumeister, R., Vohs, K., Aaker, J., & Garbinsky, E. N. (2013). Some key differences between a happy life and a meaningful life. *Journal of Positive Psychology, 8*(6, Positive Psychology in Search for Meaning), 505–516. https://doi.org/10.1080/17439 760.2013.830764

Bedaso, A., Mekonnen, N., & Duko, B. (2022). Prevalence and factors associated with preoperative anxiety among patients undergoing surgery in low-income and middle-income countries: A systematic review and meta-analysis. *BMJ Open, 12*(3). https://doi.org/10.1136/bmjopen-2021-058187

Binder, P. E. (2022). Suffering a healthy life—On the existential dimension of health. *Frontiers in Psychology, 13*, 77. https://doi.org/10.3389/fpsyg.2022.803792

Binswanger, L. (1963). Being-in-the-World: Selected Papers of Ludwig Binswanger. Basic Books.

Bishop, F. L., Lauche, R., Cramer, H., Pinto, J. W., Leung, B., Hall, H., Leach, M., Chung, V. C. H., Sundberg, T., Zhang, Y., Steel, A., Ward, L., Sibbritt, D., & Adams, J. (2019). Health behavior change and complementary medicine use: National Health Interview Survey 2012. *Medicina, 55*(10), 632. https://doi.org/10.3390/MEDICINA55100632

Böhmer, M. C., La Cour, P., & Schnell, T. (2022). A randomized controlled trial of the sources of meaning card method: A new meaning-oriented approach predicts depression, anxiety, pain acceptance, and crisis of meaning in patients with chronic pain. *Pain Medicine (United States), 23*(2), 314–325. https://doi.org/10.1093/pm/pnab321

Bolton, D., & Gillett, G. (2019). *The biopsychosocial model of health and disease: New philosophical and scientific developments.* Palgrave Macmillan.

Borrell-Carrió, F., Suchman, A. L., & Epstein, R. M. (2004). The biopsychosocial model 25 years later: Principles, practice, and scientific inquiry. *Annals of Family Medicine, 2*(6), 576–582. https://doi.org/10.1370/afm.245

Braam, a W., Van den Eeden, P., Prince, M. J., Beekman, A. T. F., Kivelä, S.-L. L., Lawlor, B. a, Birkhofer, A., Fuhrer, R., Lobo, a, Magnusson, H., Mann, a H., Meller, I., Roelands, M., Skoog, I., Turrina, C., & Copeland, J. R. M. (2001). Religion as a cross-cultural determinant of depression in elderly Europeans: results from the EURODEP collaboration. Psychological Medicine, *31*(5), 803–814. https://doi.org/10.1017/S00332 91701003956

Brayne, A. B., Brayne, R. P., & Fowler, A. J. (2021). Medical specialties and life expectancy: An analysis of doctors' obituaries 1997–2019. *Lifestyle Medicine, 2*(1), e23. https://doi.org/10.1002/LIM2.23

Brodersen, J., Siersma, V., & Ryle, M. (2011). Breast cancer screening: ' "reassuring" ' the worried well? *Scandinavian Journal of Public Health, 39*(3), 326–332. https://doi.org/10.1177/1403494810396558

Brodsky, N., Ames, A., Brown, T., & Finley, P. (2011). *Application of complex adaptive systems of systems engineering to tobacco products.* www.osti.gov/servlets/purl/1106896

Brooker, D. (2004). What is person-centred care in dementia? *Reviews in Clinical Gerontology, 13*(3), 215–222. https://doi.org/10.1017/S095925980400108X

Cao, X., & Ji, S. (2024). Bidirectional relationship between self-rated health and the big five personality traits among Chinese adolescents: A two-wave cross-lagged study. *Humanities and Social Sciences Communications, 11*(1), 1–11. https://doi.org/10.1057/s41599-024-02699-x

Capra, F. (2015). The systems view of life a unifying conception of mind, matter, and life. *Cosmos and History, 11*(2), 242–249. http://cosmosandhistory.org/index.php/journal/article/view/503

Card, A. J. (2023). The biopsychosociotechnical model: A systems-based framework for human-centered health improvement. *Health Systems, 12*(4), 387–407. https://doi.org/10.1080/20476965.2022.2029584

Carriere, K. R. (2014). Culture cultivating culture: The four products of the meaning-made world. *Integrative Psychological and Behavioral Science, 48*(3), 270–282. https://doi.org/10.1007/s12124-013-9252-0

Cameron, L., Lawler, S., Robbins-Hill, A., Toor, I., & Brown, P. (2023). Political views, health literacy, and COVID-19 beliefs and behaviors: a moderated mediation model. *Social Science & Medicine, 320*(115672). https://doi.org/10.1016/j.socscimed.2023.115672

Chida, Y., Steptoe, A., & Powell, L. H. (2009). Religiosity/spirituality and mortality. A systematic quantitative review. *Psychotherapy and Psychosomatics, 78*(2), 81–90. https://doi.org/10.1159/000190791

Claridge, T. (2020). *Current definitions of social capital: Academic definitions in 2019.* www.mendeley.com/catalogue/635ab274-439c-3131-b602-8820954e6044/?utm_source=desktop&utm_medium=1.19.8&utm_campaign=open_catalog&userDocumentId=%7B7dc3b04d-c4c2-39de-b551-6612bbdd01d5%7D

Clottes, J., & Lewis-Williams, J. D. (1998). *The Shamans of prehistory: Trance and magic in the painted caves.* Harry N. Abrams.

Cohen, R., Bavishi, C., & Rozanski, A. (2015). Purpose in life and its relationship to all-cause mortality and cardiovascular events: A meta-analysis. *Circulation, 131*(Suppl_1), A52–. https://doi.org/10.1097/PSY.0000000000000274

Conner, M., & Norman, P. (2017). Health behaviour: Current issues and challenges. *Psychology and Health, 32*(8), 895–906. https://doi.org/10.1080/08870446.2017.1336240

Cooper, M. (2003). *Existential therapies.* Sage.

Cormack, B., Stilwell, P., Coninx, S., & Gibson, J. (2022). The biopsychosocial model is lost in translation: From misrepresentation to an enactive modernization. *Physiotherapy Theory and Practice, 39*(11), 2273–2288. https://doi.org/10.1080/09593985.2022.2080130

Coulter, A., & Oldham, J. (2016). Person-centred care: What is it and how do we get there? *Future Healthcare Journal, 3*(2), 114–116. https://doi.org/10.7861/futurehosp.3-2-114

Crumbaugh, J. C., & Maholick, L. T. (1964). An experimental study in existentialism: The psychometric approach to Frankl's concept of noogenic neurosis. *Journal of Clinical Psychology, 20*(2), 200–207.

Czekierda, K., Banik, A., Park, C. L., & Luszczynska, A. (2017). Meaning in life and physical health: Systematic review and meta-analysis. *Health Psychology Review, 11*(4), 387–418. https://doi.org/10.1080/17437199.2017.1327325

DeMarinis, V. (2008). The impact of postmodernization on existential health in Sweden: Psychology of religion's function in existential public health analysis. *Archive for the Psychology of Religion/Archiv Für Religionspychologie, 30*(1), 57–74.

Diener, E., Pressman, S. D., Hunter, J., & Delgadillo-Chase, D. (2017). If, why, and when subjective well-being influences health, and future needed research. *Applied Psychology: Health and Well-Being, 9*(2), 133–167. https://doi.org/10.1111/APHW.12090

Disabato, D. J., Goodman, F. R., Kashdan, T. B., Short, J. L., & Jarden, A. (2016). Different types of well-being? A cross-cultural examination of hedonic and eudaimonic well-being. *Psychological Assessment, 28*(5), 471–482. https://doi.org/10.1037/PAS0000209

Dyar, O. J., Haglund, B. J. A., Melder, C., Skillington, T., Kristenson, M., & Sarkadi, A. (2022). Rainbows over the world's public health: determinants of health models in the past, present, and future. *Scandinavian Journal of Public Health, 50*(7), 1047–1058. https://doi.org/10.1177/14034948221113147

Dyer, A. R. (2011). The need for a new "new medical model." *Southern Medical Journal, 104*(4), 297–298. https://doi.org/10.1097/SMJ.0b013e318208767b

Dyrbye, L., West, C., Johnson, P., Cipriano, P., Peterson, C., Beatty, D., Major-Elechi, B., & Shanafelt, T. (2020). Original research: An investigation of career choice regret among American nurses. *American Journal of Nursing, 120*(4), 24–33. https://doi.org/10.1097/01.NAJ.0000660020.17156.ae

Engel, G. L. (1977). The need for a new medical model: A challenge for biomedicine. *Science, 196*(4286), 129–136. www.ncbi.nlm.nih.gov/pubmed/847460

Engel, G. L. (1980). The clinical application of the biopsychosocial model. *American Journal of Psychiatry, 137*(5), 535–544. https://doi.org/10.1176/ajp.137.5.535

Eriksson, M. (2022). The sense of coherence: The concept and its relationship to health. In *The handbook of Salutogenesis* (2nd ed., pp. 61–68). https://doi.org/10.1007/978-3-030-79515-3_9

Eriksson, M., & Lindström, B. (2005). Validity of Antonovsky's sense of coherence scale: A systematic review. *Journal of Epidemiology and Community Health, 59*(6), 460–466. https://doi.org/10.1136/jech.2003.018085

Fernandes-Osterhold, G. (2021). Diversity and Inclusion in Integral Education: A Teaching Perspective of Integral Psychology: https://doi.org/10.1177/15413446211006646. https://doi.org/10.1177/15413446211006646

Ferreira, A. (2018). Towards an integrative perspective: Bringing Ken Wilber's philosophy to planning theory and practice. *Planning Theory and Practice, 19*(4), 558–577. https://doi.org/10.1080/14649357.2018.1496270

Fitchett, G., Murphy, P. E., Kim, J., Gibbons, J. L., Cameron, J. R., & Davis, J. A. (2004). Religious struggle: Prevalence, correlates and mental health risks in diabetic, congestive heart failure, and oncology patients. *International Journal of Psychiatry in Medicine, 34*(2), 179–196. www.ncbi.nlm.nih.gov/pubmed/15387401

Flensborg-Madsen, T., Ventegodt, S., & Merrick, J. (2005). Sense of coherence and physical health. A review of previous findings. *The Scientific World Journal, 5*, 665–673. https://doi.org/10.1100/TSW.2005.85

Fraser, G. E., & Shavlik, D. J. (2001). Ten years of life is it a matter of choice? *Archives of Internal Medicine, 161*(13), 1645–1652. https://doi.org/10.1001/archinte.161.13.1645

Freeman, J. (2005). Towards a definition of holism. *British Journal of General Practice, 55*(511).

Fruth, B., Ikombe, N. B., Matshimba, G. K., Metzger, S., Muganza, D. M., Mundry, R., & Fowler, A. (2014). New evidence for self-medication in bonobos: *Manniophyton fulvum* leaf- and stemstrip-swallowing from LuiKotale, Salonga National Park, DR Congo. *American Journal of Primatology, 76*(2), 146–158. https://doi.org/10.1002/AJP.22217

Gadamer, H.-G. (1993). *The enigma of health*. Polity Press.

Gadamer, H.-G. (1996). *The enigma of health*. Polity Press.

Galanis, P., Moisoglou, I., Katsiroumpa, A., Vraka, I., Siskou, O., Konstantakopoulou, O., Meimeti, E., & Kaitelidou, D. (2023). Increased job burnout and reduced job satisfaction for nurses compared to other healthcare workers after the COVID-19 pandemic. *Nursing Reports*, *13*(3), 1090–1100. https://doi.org/10.3390/nursrep13030095

Gatseva, P. D., & Argirova, M. (2011). Public health: The science of promoting health. *Journal of Public Health*, *19*(3), 205–206. https://doi.org/10.1007/S10389-011-0412-8

Geana, M. V., Rabb, N., & Sloman, S. (2021). Walking the party line: The growing role of political ideology in shaping health behavior in the United States. *SSM - Population Health*, *16*, 100950. https://doi.org/10.1016/J.SSMPH.2021.100950

Ghaemi, S. N. (2010). *The rise and fall of the biopsychosocial model: Reconciling art and science in psychiatry*. Johns Hopkins University Press.

Goodman, A. (1991). Organic unit theory: The mind-body problem revisited. *The American Journal of Psychiatry*, *148*(5), 553–563. http://search.proquest.com/openview/46a07 cae798b7a83064cd5417fb7bc82/1?pq-origsite=gscholar&cbl=40661

Greyson, B. (2022). Persistence of attitude changes after near-death experiences: Do they fade over time? *Journal of Nervous and Mental Disease*, *210*(9), 692–696. https://doi.org/10.1097/NMD.0000000000001521

Guignon C. B. (2002). Existentialism. In E. Craig (Ed.), *Routledge encyclopedia of philosophy*. Routledge.

Hardy, K. (2021). Paleomedicine and the evolutionary context of medicinal plant use. In *Revista Brasileira de Farmacognosia* (Vol. *31*, Issue 1). https://doi.org/10.1007/s43 450-020-00107-4

Haslam, S. A., Haslam, C., Jetten, J., Cruwys, T., & Bentley, S. v. (2021). Rethinking the nature of the person at the heart of the biopsychosocial model: Exploring social changeways not just personal pathways. *Social Science & Medicine*, *272*, 113566. https://doi.org/10.1016/J.SOCSCIMED.2020.113566

Hatala, A. R. (2012). The status of the "biopsychosocial" model in health psychology: Towards an integrated approach and a critique of cultural conceptions. *Open Journal of Medical Psychology*, *01*(04), 51–62. https://doi.org/10.4236/ojmp.2012.14009

Hatfield, G., & Pittman, H. (2013). *Evolution of mind, brain, and culture*. University of Pennsylvania Museum of Archaeology and Anthropology.

Hayes, S. C., Strosahl, K. D., & Wilson, K. G. (2003). *Acceptance and commitment therapy: An experiential approach to behavior change*. The Guilford Press.

Henningsen, P. (2015). Still modern? Developing the biopsychosocial model for the 21st century. *Journal of Psychosomatic Research*, *79*(5), 362–363. https://doi.org/10.1016/j.jpsychores.2015.09.003

Henriksen, J., Larsen, E., Mattisson, C., & Anderseon, N. W. (2019). Loneliness, health and mortality. *Epidemiology and Psychiatric Sciences*, *28*, 234–239. www.cambridge.org/core/journals/epidemiology-and-psychiatric-sciences/article/loneliness-health-and-mortality/56731F5EA7C83109FD6BBD7D090C2AA9

Hergenhahn, B. R. (1997). *An introduction to the history of psychology* (3rd ed.). Brooks/Cole Publishing Company.

Høffding, H. (1916). *Den store Humor. En psykologisk studie*. Gyldendalske Boghandel. Nordisk Forlag.

Hvidt, N. C., Assing Hvidt, E., & la Cour, P. (2021). Meanings of "the existential" in a secular country: A survey study. *Journal of Religion and Health*, *61*(4), 3276–3301. https://doi.org/10.1007/S10943-021-01253-2

Idler, E. L., & Benyamini, Y. (1997). Self-rated health and mortality: A review of twenty-seven community studies. *Journal of Health and Social Behavior*, *38*(1), 21–37. https://doi.org/10.2307/2955359

Illich, I. (1975). *Medical nemesis*. Pantheon Book.

Ilori, O., Kolawole, T. O., & Olaboye, J. A. (2024). Ethical dilemmas in healthcare management: A comprehensive review. *International Medical Science Research Journal*, *4*(6), 703–725. https://doi.org/10.51594/IMSRJ.V4I6.1251

Insel, P., Roth, W., Irwin, J., & Burke, S. (2011). *Core concepts in health*. McGraw-Hill. https://ir.lib.uwo.ca/healthstudiespub/26/

James, W. (1890). *The principles of psychology*. Dover Publications. http://psychclassics.yorku.ca/James/Principles/

James, W. (1902). The varieties of religious experience. In *William James. Writings 1902–1910* (1987th ed., pp. 1–479). The Library of America.

Jarden, A., & Roache, A. (2023). What is wellbeing? *International Journal of Environmental Research and Public Health*, *20*(6). https://doi.org/10.3390/IJERPH20065006

Kannan, V., & Veazie, P. J. (2018). Political orientation, political environment, and health behaviors in the United States. *Preventive Medicine*. https://doi.org/10.1016/j.ypmed.2018.06.011

Karunamuni, N., Imayama, I., & Goonetilleke, D. (2021). Pathways to well-being: Untangling the causal relationships among biopsychosocial variables. *Social Science & Medicine*, *272*, 112846. https://doi.org/10.1016/J.SOCSCIMED.2020.112846

Kashdan, T. B., & Rottenberg, J. (2010). Psychological flexibility as a fundamental aspect of health. *Clinical Psychology Review*, *30*(7), 865. https://doi.org/10.1016/J.CPR.2010.03.001

Key, T. J., Fraser, G. E., Thorogood, M., Appleby, P. N., Beral, V., Reeves, G., Burr, M. L., Chang-Claude, J., Frentzel-Beyme, R., Kuzma, J. W., Mann, J., & McPherson, K. (1999). Mortality in vegetarians and nonvegetarians: Detailed findings from a collaborative analysis of 5 prospective studies. *American Journal of Clinical Nutrition*, *70*(3 Suppl.). https://doi.org/10.1093/ajcn/70.3.516s

Keyes, K. M., & Platt, J. M. (2024). Annual research review: Sex, gender, and internalizing conditions among adolescents in the 21st century – trends, causes, consequences. *Journal of Child Psychology and Psychiatry and Allied Disciplines*, *65*(4), 384–407. https://doi.org/10.1111/jcpp.13864

Khanfar, A. N., Alshrouf, M. A., Albandi, A. M., Odeh, Q. B., Hammad, N. H., Abu Jbara, F. K., & AlRyalat, S. A. (2023). Career regret and health-related quality of life among medical students: A nationwide cross-sectional study in Jordan. *Journal of Medical Education and Curricular Development*, *10*. https://doi.org/10.1177/23821205231219428

Kishon, R., Modlin, N. L., Cycowicz, Y. M., Mourtada, H., Wilson, T., Williamson, V., Cleare, A., & Rucker, J. (2024). A rapid narrative review of the clinical evolution of psychedelic treatment in clinical trials. *Npj Mental Health Research*, *3*(1). https://doi.org/10.1038/s44184-024-00068-9

Koenig, H. G. (2000). Religion and medicine I: Historical background and reasons for separation. *International Journal of Psychiatry in Medicine*, *30*(4), 385–398. www.ncbi.nlm.nih.gov/pubmed/11308040

Koenig, H. G., Georg, L. K., & Peterson, B. L. (1998). Religiosity and remission of depression in medically ill older patients. *American Journal of Psychiatry*, *155*, 536–542.

Koenig, H., King, D., & Carson, V. B. (2012). *Handbook of religion and health*. Oxford University Press.

Kyte, L., & Wells, C. (2010). Variations in life expectancy between rural and urban areas of England, 2001-07. *Health Statistics Quarterly / Office for National Statistics*, *46*, 25–50. https://doi.org/10.1057/HSQ.2010.10

la Cour, P., Ausker, N. H., & Hvidt, N. C. (2012). Six understandings of the word spirituality in a secular country. *Archive for the Psychology of Religion/Archiv Für Religionspychologie, 34*(1), 63–81. https://doi.org/10.1163/157361212X649634.

la Cour, P., Avlund, K., & Schultz-Larsen, K. (2006). Religion and survival in a secular region. A twenty year follow-up of 734 Danish adults born in 1914. *Social Science and Medicine, 62*(1), 157–164. https://doi.org/10.1016/j.socscimed.2005.05.029

la Cour, P., & Hvidt, N. C. (2010). Research on meaning-making and health in secular society: Secular, spiritual and religious existential orientations. *Social Science & Medicine, 71*(7), 1292–1299. https://doi.org/10.1016/j.socscimed.2010.06.024

la Cour, P., & Schnell, T. (2020). Presentation of the sources of meaning card method: The SoMeCaM. *Journal of Humanistic Psychology, 60*(1), 20–42. https://doi.org/10.1177/0022167816669620

Länsimies, H., Pietilä, A. M., Hietasola-Husu, S., & Kangasniemi, M. (2017). A systematic review of adolescents' sense of coherence and health. *Scandinavian Journal of Caring Sciences, 31*(4), 651–661. https://doi.org/10.1111/SCS.12402

Larsson, H., Saarelainen, S., Sjöberg, M., Dezutter, J., & Haugan, G. (2024). Existential loneliness and meaning-in-life in the lived experience of nursing home residents. *Journal of Care and Caring*, 1–19. https://bristoluniversitypressdigital.com/view/journals/ijcc/aop/article-10.1332-23978821Y2024D000000047/article-10.1332-23978821Y2024D000000047.xml

Lehman, B. J., David, D. M., & Gruber, J. A. (2017). Rethinking the biopsychosocial model of health: Understanding health as a dynamic system. *Social and Personality Psychology Compass, 11*(8), 1–17. https://doi.org/10.1111/spc3.12328

Lind, A. B., Risoer, M. B., Nielsen, K., Delmar, C., Christensen, M. B., & Lomborg, K. (2014). Longing for existential recognition: A qualitative study of everyday concerns for people with somatoform disorders. *Journal of Psychosomatic Research, 76*(2), 99–104. https://doi.org/10.1016/j.jpsychores.2013.11.005

Lindström, M., Pirouzifard, M., Rosvall, M., & Fridh, M. (2022). Health locus of control and all-cause, cardiovascular, cancer and other cause mortality: A population-based prospective cohort study in southern Sweden. *Preventive Medicine, 161*. https://doi.org/10.1016/j.ypmed.2022.107114

Liu, H., Liu, N., Chong, S. T., Boon Yau, E. K., & Ahmad Badayai, A. R. (2023). Effects of acceptance and commitment therapy on cognitive function: A systematic review. *Heliyon, 9*(3), e14057. https://doi.org/10.1016/j.heliyon.2023.e14057

Luo, Y., Hawkley, L. C., Waite, L. J., & Cacioppo, J. T. (2012). Loneliness, health, and mortality in old age: A national longitudinal study. *Social Science and Medicine, 74*(6), 907–914. https://doi.org/10.1016/j.socscimed.2011.11.028

Marks, D., Murray, M., & Estacio, E. V. (2018). *Health psychology: Theory, research and practice* (5th ed.). Sage.

Martin, S. C., & Howell, J. D. (1989). One hundred years of clinical preventive medicine in America. *Primary Care – Clinics in Office Practice, 16*(1), 3–8+vii. https://doi.org/10.1016/s0095-4543(21)01305-1

Marulappa, N., Anderson, N. N., Bethell, J., Bourbonnais, A., Kelly, F., McMurray, J., Rogers, H. L., Vedel, I., & Gagliardi, A. R. (2022). How to implement person-centred care and support for dementia in outpatient and home/community settings: Scoping review. *BMC Health Services Research, 22*(1). https://doi.org/10.1186/s12913-022-07875-w

McLaren, N. (1998). A critical review of the biopsychosocial model. *Australian and New Zealand Journal of Psychiatry, 32*, 86–92.

Melder, C. (2012). The epidemiology of lost meaning: A study in the psychology of religion and existential public health. *Scripta Instituti Donneriani Aboensis, 2012*. https://journal.fi/scripta/article/view/67417

Melder, C. (2022). Existential public health and existential care in secular and interfaith contexts. In *Complexities of spiritual care in plural societies* (pp. 162–191). www.degruyter.com/document/doi/10.1515/9783110717365/pdf#page=197

Mendes, M., Simões, P. A., Simões, J. A., Santiago, L. M., Prazeres, F., & Maricoto, T. (2023). The link between happiness and health: A review of concepts, pathways and strategies for enhancing well-being. *Family Medicine and Primary Care Review, 25*(3), 288–296. https://doi.org/10.5114/fmpcr.2023.130090

Michaelson, J., Mahony, S., & Schifferes, J. (2012). *Measuring wellbeing: A guide for practitioners*. New Economics Foundation.

Mirdal, G. M. (1990). *Psykosomatik*. Munksgaard.

Mitchell, J. M., & Anderson, B. T. (2023). Psychedelic therapies reconsidered: Compounds, clinical indications, and cautious optimism. *Neuropsychopharmacology, 49*(1), 96–103. https://doi.org/10.1038/s41386-023-01656-7

Modig, K., Talbäck, M., Torssander, J., & Ahlbom, A. (2017). Payback time? Influence of having children on mortality in old age. *Journal of Epidemiology and Community Health, 71*(5), 424–430. https://doi.org/10.1136/JECH-2016-207857

Molina, J. A. (1984). Understanding the biopsychosocial model. *The International Journal of Psychiatry in Medicine, 13*(1), 29–36. https://doi.org/10.2190/0UHQ-BXNE-6GGY-N1TF

Moreira-Almeida, A., & Koenig, H. G. (2006). Retaining the meaning of the words religiousness and spirituality: A commentary on the WHOQOL SRPB group's "cross-cultural study of spirituality, religion, and personal beliefs as components of quality of life". *Social Science & Medicine, 63*(4), 843–845. https://doi.org/10.1016/j.socscimed.2006.03.001

Musich, S., Wang, S., Kraemer, S., Hawkins, K., & Wicker, E. (2018). Purpose in life and positive health outcomes among older adults. *Liebertpub.Com, 21*(2), 139–147. https://doi.org/10.1089/pop.2017.0063

Nahin, R. L., Feinberg, T., Kapos, F. P., & Terman, G. W. (2023). Estimated rates of incident and persistent chronic pain among US adults, 2019–2020. *JAMA Network Open, 6*(5), e2313563. https://doi.org/10.1001/JAMANETWORKOPEN.2023.13563

Neco, L. C., Abelson, E. S., Brown, A., Natterson-Horowitz, B., & Blumstein, D. T. (2019). The evolution of self-medication behaviour in mammals. *Biological Journal of the Linnean Society, 128*(2), 373–378. https://doi.org/10.1093/biolinnean/blz117

Nygaard, M. R., Austad, A., Sørensen, T., Synnes, O., & McSherry, W. (2022). 'Existential' in Scandinavian healthcare journals: An analysis of the concept and implications for future research. *Religions, 13*(10). https://doi.org/10.3390/rel13100979

Ogden, J. (2012). *Health psychology. A textbook* (5th ed.). Open University Press. www.google.com/books?hl=da&lr=&id=RzVFBgAAQBAJ&oi=fnd&pg=PR1&dq=jane+odgen&ots=JyJpVjTiQt&sig=OD67V56MF3KUYvZmMrexZUjhxBE

Pandey, S., & Sharma, V. (2019). Doctor, heal thyself: Addressing the shorter life expectancy of doctors in India. *Indian Journal of Ophthalmology, 67*(7), 1248–1250. https://doi.org/10.4103/ijo.IJO_656_19

Pargament, K. I., Koenig, H. G., Tarakeshwar, N., & Hahn, J. (2001). Religious struggle as a predictor of mortality among medically ill elderly patients. A 2-year longitudinal study. *Archives of Internal Medicine, 161*, 1881–1885.

Park, K. (1994). The criminal and the saintly body: Autopsy and dissection in Renaissance Italy. *Renaissance Quarterly, 47*(1), 1–33. www.cambridge.org/core/journals/renaissa nce-quarterly/article/criminal-and-the-saintly-body-autopsy-and-dissection-in-renaissa nce-italy/7A109F43AA3900298D626DE70CD47B19

Pehlivanova, M., Carroll, A., & Greyson, B. (2023). Which near-death experience features are associated with reduced fear of death? *Mortality, 28*(3), 493–509. https://doi.org/ 10.1080/13576275.2021.2017868

Peng-Keller, S., Winiger, F., & Rauch, R. (2022). *The spirit of global health: The World Health Organization and the "spiritual dimension" of health, 1946–2021.* Oxford University Press. 10.1093/oso/9780192865502.001.0001.

Phyo, A. Z. Z., Freak-Poli, R., Craig, H., Gasevic, D., Stocks, N. P., Gonzalez-Chica, D. A., & Ryan, J. (2020). Quality of life and mortality in the general population: A systematic review and meta-analysis. *BMC Public Health, 20*(1). https://doi.org/10.1186/S12 889-020-09639-9

Pigliucci, M. (2008). The borderlands between science and philosophy: An introduction. *Quarterly Review of Biology, 83*(1), 7–15. https://doi.org/10.1086/529558

Pilgrim, D. (2002). The biopsychosocial model in Anglo-American psychiatry: Past, present and future? *Journal of Mental Health, 11*(6), 585–594. https://doi.org/10.1080/096382 30020023930

Pomerleau, O. F., & Brady, J. P. (1979). *Behavioral medicine, theory and practice.* Williams & Wilkins.

Porter, R. (2003). *Medicinens historie.* Rosinante.

Pretty, J., & Ward, H. (2001). Social capital and the environment. *World Development, 29*(2), 209–227. https://doi.org/10.1016/S0305-750X(00)00098-X

Prochaska, J. O., & Velicer, W. F. (1997). The transtheoretical model of health behavior change. *American Journal of Health Promotion, 12*(1), 38–48. https://doi.org/10.4278/ 0890-1171-12.1.38

Reinwarth, A. C., Wicke, F. S., Hettich, N., Ernst, M., Otten, D., Brähler, E., Wild, P. S., Münzel, T., König, J., Lackner, K. J., Pfeiffer, N., & Beutel, M. E. (2023). Self-rated physical health predicts mortality in aging persons beyond objective health risks. *Scientific Reports, 13*(1). https://doi.org/10.1038/s41598-023-46882-7

Rico-Uribe, L. A., Caballero, F. F., Martín-María, N., Cabello, M., Ayuso-Mateos, J. L., & Miret, M. (2018). Association of loneliness with all-cause mortality: A meta-analysis. *PLoS ONE, 13*(1). https://doi.org/10.1371/JOURNAL.PONE.0190033

Robles, T. F. (2014). Marital quality and health: Implications for marriage in the 21st century. *Current Directions in Psychological Science, 23*(6), 427. https://doi.org/10.1177/09637 21414549043

Robles, T. F., Slatcher, R. B., Trombello, J. M., & McGinn, M. M. (2014). Marital quality and health: A meta-analytic review. *Psychological Bulletin, 140*(1), 140–187. https://doi. org/10.1037/A0031859

Roepke, A. M., Jayawickreme, E., & Riffle, O. M. (2014). Meaning and health: A systematic review. *Applied Research in Quality of Life, 9*(4), 1055–1079. https://doi.org/10.1007/ S11482-013-9288-9

Rogers, N. T., Demakakos, P., Taylor, M. S., Steptoe, A., Hamer, M., & Shankar, A. (2016). Volunteering is associated with increased survival in able-bodied participants of the English Longitudinal Study of Ageing. *Journal of Epidemiology and Community Health, 70*(6), 583. https://doi.org/10.1136/JECH-2015-206305

Rovner, B. W. (1991). Depression and mortality. *JAMA: The Journal of the American Medical Association, 265*(8), 993. https://doi.org/10.1001/jama.1991.03460080063033

Rowe-Johnson, M. K., Browning, B., & Scott, B. (2024). Effects of acceptance and commitment therapy on trauma-related symptoms: A systematic review and meta-analysis. *Psychological Trauma: Theory, Research, Practice, and Policy.* https://doi.org/10.1037/tra0001785

Ryff, C. D., & Singer, B. H. (2008). Know thyself and become what you are: A eudaimonic approach to psychological well-being. *Journal of Happiness Studies, 9*(1), 13–39. https://doi.org/10.1007/s10902-006-9019-0

Salander, P. (2006). Who needs the concept of 'spirituality'? *Psychooncology, 15*(7), 647–649.

Sand, L., & Strang, P. (2006). Existential loneliness in a palliative home care setting. *Journal of Palliative Medicine, 9*(6), 1376–1387. https://doi.org/10.1089/JPM.2006.9.1376

Schnell, T. (2009). The sources of meaning and meaning in life questionnaire (SoMe): Relations to demographics and well-being. *The Journal of Positive Psychology, 4*(6), 483–499. https://doi.org/10.1080/17439760903271074

Schnell, T. (2011). Individual differences in meaning-making: Considering the variety of sources of meaning, their density and diversity. *Personality and Individual Differences, 51*(5), 667–673.

Schnell, T. (2021). *The psychology of meaning in life.* Routledge.

Sebo, P., Tudrej, B., Bernard, A., Delaunay, B., Dupuy, A., Malavergne, C., & Maisonneuve, H. (2024). Validation and refinement of the sense of coherence scale for a French population: Observational study. *Interactive Journal of Medical Research, 13*, e50284. https://doi.org/10.2196/50284

Sejrsgaard, M., Hvidtjørn, D., & Prinds, C. (2024). The paradox of awareness of death in parenthood transition—A qualitative study. *Death Studies.* https://doi.org/10.1080/07481187.2024.2361744

Shah, R., & Foell, J. (2023). *Fighting for the soul of General practice. The algorithm will see you now.* Intellect.

Sigurdson, O. (2016). Existential health. Philosophical and historical perspectives. *LIR Journal, 6*(16), 7–23.

Sigurdson, O. (2019). Only vulnerable creatures suffer: On suffering, embodiment and existential health. In E. Dahl, C. Falke, & T. E. eriksen (Eds.), *Phenomenology of the broken body.* Routledge. www.taylorfrancis.com/chapters/edit/10.4324/9780429462542-6/vulnerable-creatures-suffer-ola-sigurdson

Smith, C., & Davidson, H. (2014). *The paradox of generosity: Giving we receive, grasping we lose.* www.google.com/books?hl=da&lr=&id=QGvrAwAAQBAJ&oi=fnd&pg=PP1&dq=generosity+health+review+blood&ots=3nX1VsvFA-&sig=vDVgZsVbs1eafOtyD5uJCTDmlYs

Smith, R. C. (2021). Making the biopsychosocial model more scientific-its general and specific models. *Social Science & Medicine, 272*, 113568. https://doi.org/10.1016/j.socscimed.2020.113568

Spinelli, E. (2005). *The interpreted world: An introduction to phenomenological psychology.* Sage.

Spinelli, E. (2014). Practising existential psychotherapy. The relational world. วารสารวิชาการมหาวิทยาลัยอีสเทิร์นเอเชีย, *4*(1). Sage Publications. www.torrossa.com/gs/resourceProxy?an=5019121&publisher=FZ7200

Stacey, D., Paquet, L., & Samant, R. (2010). Exploring cancer treatment decision-making by patients: A descriptive study. *Current Oncology*, *17*(4), 85–93. https://doi.org/10.3747/co.v17i4.527

Steffler, M., Li, Y., Weir, S., Shaikh, S., Murtada, F., Wright, J. G., & Kantarevic, J. (2021). Trends in prevalence of chronic disease and multimorbidity in Ontario, Canada. *CMAJ*, *193*(8), E270–E277. https://doi.org/10.1503/cmaj.201473

Steger, M., Frazier, P., Oishi, S., & Kaler, M. (2006). The meaning in life questionnaire: Assessing the presence of and search for meaning in life. *Journal of Counseling Psychology*. https://doi.org/10.1037/0022-0167.53.1.80

Stenlund, S., Koivumaa-Honkanen, H., Sillanmäki, L., Lagström, H., Rautava, P., & Suominen, S. (2022). Changed health behavior improves subjective well-being and vice versa in a follow -up of 9 years. *Health and Quality of Life Outcomes*, *20*(1), 1–12. https://doi.org/10.1186/s12955-022-01972-4

Steptoe, A. (2019). Happiness and health. *Annual Review of Public Health*, *40*, 339–359. https://doi.org/10.1146/ANNUREV-PUBLHEALTH-040218-044150

Strang, P. (1997). Existential consequences of unrelieved cancer pain. *Palliative Medicine*, *11*(4), 299–305. https://doi.org/10.1177/026921639701100406

Strang, P. (2014). What is extreme death anxiety and what are its consequences? *Journal of Palliative Care*, *30*(4), 321–326. https://doi.org/10.1177/082585971403000416

Strang, P., Strang, S., Hultborn, R., & Arner, S. (2004). Existential pain—an entity, a provocation, or a challenge? *Journal of Pain and Symptom Management*, *27*(3), 241–250. www.sciencedirect.com/science/article/pii/S0885392403005165

Szcześniak, M., Świątek, A. H., Cieślak, M., & Świdurska, D. (2020). Disease acceptance and eudemonic well-being among adults with physical disabilities: The mediator effect of meaning in life. *Frontiers in Psychology*, *11*, 525560. doi.org/10.3389/fpsyg.2020.525560

Tavakoli, H. R. (2009). A closer evaluation of current methods in psychiatric assessments: A challenge for the biopsychosocial model. *Psychiatry* (Edgmont (Pa.: Township)), *6*(2), 25–30.

Valtonen, J., Ilmarinen, V. J., & Lönnqvist, J. E. (2023). Political orientation predicts the use of conventional and complementary/alternative medicine: A survey study of 19 European countries. *Social Science and Medicine*, *331*, 116089. https://doi.org/10.1016/j.socscimed.2023.116089

Van Deurzen, E., & Arnold-Baker, C. (2005). *Existential perspectives on human issues: A handbook for therapeutic practice*. Palgrave Macmillan.

von dem Knesebeck, O., Verde, P. E., & Dragano, N. (2006). Education and health in 22 European countries. *Social Science and Medicine*, *63*(5), 1344–1351. https://doi.org/10.1016/j.socscimed.2006.03.043

Vowles, K., Eccleston, C., McLeod, C., & McCracken, L. (2009). Exploratory and confirmatory factor analysis of the Chronic Pain Acceptance Questionnaire. *Journal of Pain*, *10*(4S), 10.

Wagner, J., Orth, U., Bleidorn, W., Hopwood, C. J., & Kandler, C. (2020). Toward an integrative model of sources of personality stability and change. *Current Directions in Psychological Science*, *29*(5), 438–444. https://doi.org/10.1177/0963721420924751

Walker, B. H., & Brown, D. C. (2022). Trends in lifespan variation across the spectrum of rural and urban places in the United States, 1990–2017. *SSM – Population Health*, *19*. https://doi.org/10.1016/J.SSMPH.2022.101213

Walker, M., Duggan, G., Roulston, N., Van Slack, A., & Mason, G . (2012). Negative affective states and their effects on morbidity, mortality and longevity. *Animal Welfare*, *21*, 497–509. https://doi.org/10.7120/09627286.21.4.497

Wedding, D., & Stuber, M. (2020). *Behavior and medicine*. Hogrefe. www.google.com/books?hl=da&lr=&id=tp2bEAAAQBAJ&oi=fnd&pg=PR5&dq=behavior+and+medicine+wedding&ots=vW__lALkIb&sig=0_Cdy3AQuFDXtZSUHmUSaBiOMko

Whitehead, P. (2019). *Existential health psychology: The blind-spot in healthcare*. Palgrave Macmillan. www.google.com/books?hl=da&lr=&id=qAGfDwAAQBAJ&oi=fnd&pg=PR6&dq=existential+health+psychology&ots=7B0g3BXOVb&sig=vF3QHUB8R8Cwz5IE7RzTE6o3gkI

WHO. (1984). *Health promotion: A discussion document on the concept and principles: Summary report of the Working Group on Concept and Principles of Health Promotion, Copenhagen, 9–13 July 1984* (p. 8). WHO Regional Office for Europe. https://iris.who.int E90607

WHO. (2005). *Promoting mental health: Concepts, emerging evidence, practice*. www.who.int/publications/i/item/9241562943

WHO. (2022). *Mental health*. www.who.int/en/news-room/fact-sheets/detail/mental-health-strengthening-our-response

WHO. (2023). *Infertility prevalence estimates, 1990–2021*. Licence: CC BY-NC-SA 3.0 IGO. www.who.int/publications/i/item/9789240068315

WHO. (2024). *Public health and environment*. www.who.int/data/gho/data/themes/public-health-and-environment

Wilber, K. (2007). *A brief history of everything*. Shambhala.

Willroth, E. C., Ong, A. D., Graham, E. K., & Mroczek, D. K. (2020). Being happy and becoming happier as independent predictors of physical health and mortality. *Psychosomatic Medicine*, *82*(7), 650–657. https://doi.org/10.1097/PSY.0000000000000832

Yalom, I. D. (1980). *Existential psychotherapy*. Basic Books.

Zajacova, A., & Lawrence, E. M. (2018). The relationship between education and health: Reducing disparities through a contextual approach. *Annual Review of Public Health*, *39*, 273–289. https://doi.org/10.1146/ANNUREV-PUBLHEALTH-031816-044628

Zhao, B., Wang, Q., Wang, L., Chen, J., Yin, T., Zhang, J., Cheng, X., & Hou, R. (2023). Effect of acceptance and commitment therapy for depressive disorders: A meta-analysis. *Annals of General Psychiatry*, *22*(1), 34. https://doi.org/10.1186/S12991-023-00462-1

Zingmark, H., & Granberg-Axèll, A. (2022). Near-death experiences and the change of worldview in survivors of sudden cardiac arrest: A phenomenological and hermeneutical study. *Qualitative Research in Medicine & Healthcare*, *6*(3). https://doi.org/10.4081/QRMH.2022.10241

INDEX

Note: Page numbers in *italic* indicate figures and in **bold** indicate tables.

Abbas, S. Q. 95
abortion 49, 91
Acceptance and Commitment movement of
    psychotherapy (ACT) 86, 87
acceptance of suffering 86
Ahn, A. C. 36
Als, Heidelise 39
angst 57
anti-smoking campaigns 48, 96–97
Antonovsky, Aaron 83–84
anxiety, existential 57
Argirova, M. 15
artificial insemination 90
artificial intelligence (AI) 34
assisted suicide 12, 79, 80–81
Augustine 4, **6**, 43–44
authentic life 57

Barth, Karl **6**
Batson, Daniel 13–14
behavioural medicine 95
Berkeley, George **42**
Binder, Per-Einar 63–64
Binswanger, Ludwig 45
bio/body dimension of health and illness
    47, **50**
biopsychosocial (BPS) model 8, 18–31, 38;
    early critique 20–22, 32; later critique
    24–30, *27*, 32–33, 40; overlapping
    circles illustrations 22–24, *23*;
    presentation of 18–20, *19*
body–mind dualism *see* mind–body dualism
Böhmer, M. C. 86–87

Bolton, Derek 27–28, 32, 39
Borrell-Carrió, Fransesc 22, 32
British School of Existential Analysis 63
Brodsky, N. 29
Buddha 41
burials with burial gifts 3–4, 55

cancer 25, 37, 38, 47, 48, **50**, 51, 80, 92,
    93, 96, 100
Card, Alan 29–30, 33
causality *see* illness causality
childbirth 91
Christianity 4, **6**, 55–56, 77
chronic illnesses 36–37, 65, 86, 93
chronic pain 30, 61, 86–87, 93
Chronic Pain Acceptance Questionnaire 86
church attendance 77–78
climate change 16
cognitive revolution 4
cognitive/behavioural perspectives 14–15,
    48, **50**, 96
Cohen, R. 82–83
collectivist perspective 57
complementary/alternative medicine
    (CAM) 79, 87
complex adaptive system of systems
    (CASoS) 29
consciousness 40, **42**, 43, 45, 70
contextual attitude 99
Cooper, Mick 58
Cormack, Ben 30, 33
Covid-19 pandemic 35, 78–79, 91, 96, 102
culture 4, 51

death 12, 34, 35, 49, 57, 62, 63, 72, 91,
    94–95, 103; *see also* near-death
    experience; suicide
Dein, S. 95
DeMarinis, Valerie 59–60
dementia 11, 35, 94, 99
deontological perspectives 33–34
Descartes, René 5, **6**, 41
dialectic materialism **42**
disabilities 91
dissection 41
Down syndrome 99
dualism *see* mind–body dualism
Dyer, Allen 25–26, 32

education, health and 79
emergence concept 21, 38
end-of-life care 9, 64, 94–95, 99, 100
Engel, Georg L. 8, 18–20, *19*, 25, 32, 38,
    40
environmental health *see* social/
    environmental health
eudaimonic life attitude 97
eudaimonic well-being 8, 76
'existential', new understandings of 58–59
existential anxiety 57
existential expressions 72, **73**, 76–81;
    happiness and health 76–77; life
    decisions and health 79–81; personality
    traits and health 81; political orientation
    and health 78–79, 87; religion and health
    77–78
existential givens 62–64
existential guilt 57
existential health: associations 66–67;
    contextually and empirically defined
    64–66; examples during the lifespan
    90–95; in four-dimensional model
    49, **50**, 51; implications of 98–102; as
    meaning-making 59–60; prevention of
    illness and 95–97; as pure subjectivity
    60–62; in pyramid of health as a resource
    103, *104*; as reflecting the 'existential
    givens' 62–64
existential health elements 68–74, *69*,
    73; *see also* existential expressions;
    existential qualities; experience of living;
    life orientations
existential health psychology 31, 62
existential loneliness 64, 65
existential pain 64
existential phenomenology 62, 63
existential philosophy 55–58, 65
existential psychotherapy 56, 62–63, 100

existential qualities 71–72, **73**, 81–85;
    locus of control and health 84–85;
    loneliness and health 85; meaning and
    health 81–82; purpose in life and health
    82–83; quality of life and health 84;
    sense of coherence and health 83–84
experience of living 70–71, **73**, 87–89;
    near-death experience and health 88–89;
    self-rated health 88

Feuerbach, Ludwig **42**
first-person perspectives in medicine
    24–26, 30–31, 40, 49
flexibility/rigidity, psychological 87
Foell, J. 33–34
four-dimensional model of health
    and illness 46–52, *47*; abilities and
    limitations of model 51–52; bio/body
    dimension 47, **50**; cognitive/behavioural
    dimension 48, **50**; existential/
    experiential dimension 49, **50**, 52; social/
    environmental dimension 47–48, **50**
free will 57, 92

Gadamer, Hans-Georg 30–31, 61
Galen 4
Gatseva, P. D. 15
generosity 72, 81
Ghaemi, S. Nassir 18, 24–25, 32
Gillett, Grant 27–28, 32, 39
good life 49, 58, 59, 97, 98, 103
Goodman, A. 21, 32
Grinker, Roy 24–25
Groff, Stanislav **42**
guilt, existential 57

happiness 72; health and 76–77
Haslam, S. A. 29
health behaviours 78, 85–86, 95–97, 99
health literacy 78–79, 95
health policy 33, 35
health professionals: assisted suicide and
    81; life expectancy 79–80; meaning in
    work 101–102; training 100–101
health promotion 10, 95
health psychology 95; *see also* existential
    health psychology
health understandings and definitions:
    health as a resource 10–11, 12, 61, 75,
    103, *104*; health as well-being 7–8, 61,
    75; lost sense of wholeness 3–7, *5*, **6**;
    mental health 5–6, **6**, 12–15; physical
    health 11–12; social health 15–16;
    'spiritual dimension' of health 8–9;

WHO's history of defining health 7–11, 12–13, 16, 61
healthcare choices 92–93
hedonistic life attitude 97
hedonistic well-being 8, 76
Heidegger, Martin 62
Henningsen, Peter 26, 32
Hippocrates **6**
Hobbes, Thomas 21, **42**
Høffding, Harald 43
holism, defining 7
homeostasis 12, 36, 39, 47, 72
human reality, dimensions of 43–45, *44*; *see also* four-dimensional model of health and illness
humanism 14–15, 21, 25, 33–34, 49, **50**, 51, 94
Husserl, Edmund **42**, 56
Hvidt, N. C. 58, 59

ideographic perspectives 14–15
Illich, Ivan 61
illness causality 22, 24, 26, 27–28, 29, 37–40, 52
individualistic perspective 56
infertility 90
integrated model of health 32–45; dimensions of human reality 43–45, *44*; illness causality and systems theory 37–40, *39*; mind–body problem 40–43, **42**; need for in general practice 33–34; need for in health policy 35; reductionism and 35–37; *see also* four-dimensional model of health and illness

James, William 14, 43, 44
Jarden, A. 8
Jung, Carl G. **42**

Karunamuni, Nandini 28–29, 30, 32, 51
Kierkegaard, Søren 56
Koenig, Harold 77

Larsson, H. 64
Lehman, B. J. 26–27, *27*, 32
Leibniz, Gottfried 21, **42**
Leontiev, Aleksej **42**
Life Changes Inventory 88
life decisions 72; health and 79–81, 97
life expectancy 12, 78, 79–80, 86, 96
life orientations 70, 71, **73**, 85–87; basic acceptance and health 86; flexibility/rigidity and health 87; health behaviours

78, 85–86, 95–97, 99; sources of meaning and health 86–87
life philosophy 72, 78, 97
Lindström, M. 84–85
lived meaning 74
locus of control 84–85
loneliness: existential 64, 65; health and 85

McLaren, N. 21, 32
marriage, health and 80
Marx, Karl **42**
material Self 44
materialism 21, **42**
meaning in life 64, 70–71, 72, 74, 93, 100; health and 81–82, 86–87
meaning in work 101–102
meaninglessness 49, 63, 65
meaning-making 63, 65, 71; existential health as 59–60
mechanical materialism **42**
medical causality *see* illness causality
medical decision-making 92–93
medical professionals *see* health professionals
medical reductionism 35–37
medicalization of everyday life 31, 61–62, 63–64
Melder, Cecilia 60
Mendes, M. 76
mental health: crisis in young people 35, 91; defining 5–6, **6**, 12–15; existential givens and 62–63; in four-dimensional model 48, **50**; in pyramid of health as a resource 103, *104*
Merleau-Ponty, Maurice 30
Michaelson, J. 8
mind–body dualism 4–6, **6**, 21, 22, 28, 30, 40–43, **42**, 52
Mirdal, Gretty 39
models of health *see* biopsychosocial (BPS) model; four-dimensional model of health and illness; integrated model of health
Molina, J. A. 20
mono-causality 37–38, 52
Musich, S. 83

narrative medicine 41, 62
Neanderthals 3, 4
near-death experience 88–89
nomothetic perspectives 14–15, 33–34
Nygaard, Marianne Rodriguez 65–66

objective idealism **42**
Old Testament 4, **6**
Osler, William 25, 99

pain: chronic 30, 61, 86–87, 93; existential 64
palliative care 9, 64, 99, 100
Peng-Keller, S. 7, 8–9
personality traits 72; health and 81
person-centred care 94, 99
phenomenology 30–31, 44, 49; existential 62, 63; phenomenological method 56, 63
physical health: defining 11–12; in four-dimensional model 47, **50**; in pyramid of health as a resource 103, *104*
Pilgrim, David 21
Plato 4, **6**, 41
political orientation 72; health and 78–79, 87
Porter, Roy 12
pragmatic dualism 52
pre-surgery anxiety 91–92
preventative medicine 95–97
profession choice, health and 79–80
psychedelic therapy 88–89
psyche–soma relations 4–6, **6**, 21, 22, 28, 30, 40–43, **42**, 52
psychological flexibility/rigidity 87
psychosomatics 18, 25
public health 6, **6**, 15–16, 33, 37, 59–60, 95–97
pure Ego 44
purpose in life 82–83

quality of life 71, 84, 93

reductionism, medical 35–37
religion 4, **6**, 9, 55–56, 58–59, 65, 77, 86; health and 77–78; *see also* spirituality
risk factors 26, 36, 37–38, 48
Roache, A. 8
Roepke, A. M. 82, 83
Rosenberg, C. 7
Rotter, Julian 84

Salander, Pär 59
Schnell, Tatjana 72, 100, 101–102
Schoenrade, Patricia 13–14
self-rated health 88
self-transcendence 102
sense of coherence 83–84
sense of meaning 72
Seventh-Day Adventists 86
SF36 questionnaire 84, 88
Shah, R. 33–34

shamans 4, *5*, **6**
shared medical decision-making 92–93
Sigurdson, Ola 60–61
Smith, R. C. 29
smoking 37, 38, 48, 78, 85, 96–97
social capital 15
social Self 44
social/environmental health: defining 15–16; in four-dimensional model 47–48, **50**; in pyramid of health as a resource 103, *104*
Socratic dialogue 101
solipsism **42**
sources of meaning 71, 74, 100; health and 86–87
Sources of Meaning Card Method 100
Spinelli, Ernesto 56, 63
Spinoza, Baruch 21
spiritual Self 44
spirituality 8–9, 25–26, 58–59, 65, 78
Stages of Change Model 96–97
Steptoe, A. 76
Stone Age 4
Strang, Peter 64
subjective experience of living 70–71, **73**, 87–89; near-death experience and health 88–89; self-rated health 88
subjective idealism **42**
suffering 40, 49, 57, 61–62, 64, 65, 70, 93; acceptance of 86
suicide 79, 80; assisted 12, 79, 80–81; prevention services 94
surgery 91–92
systems theory 19–20, *19*, 26–30, *27*, 36, 37–40

Tavakoli, Hamid 22

Van Deurzen-Smith, Emmy 45, 63
vegetarianism 85–86
Ventis, W. Larry 13–14

well-being: defining 8; eudaimonic 8, 76; health as 7–8, 61, 75; hedonistic 8, 76
Whitehead, Patrick 31, 61–62
WHO 7–11, 12–13, 16, 60, 61, 90
wholeness of health, lost sense of 3–7, *5*, **6**
Wilber, Ken 44–45, *44*
Wundt, Wilhelm 14

Yalom, Irvin 56, 62–63